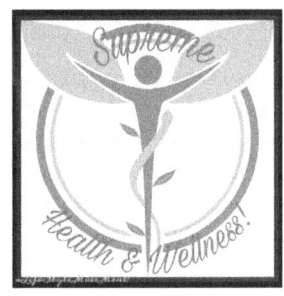

Oxygen!

*The Breath Of LIFE In Atomic Form!

Supreme Health	Kareem Tyree	Gabriella Monique
Staff & Scientist:	Khalil Malik	Sean Ali

OxyGen ... The Breath Of Life In Atomic Form!

OxyGen ... The Breath Of Life In Atomic Form!

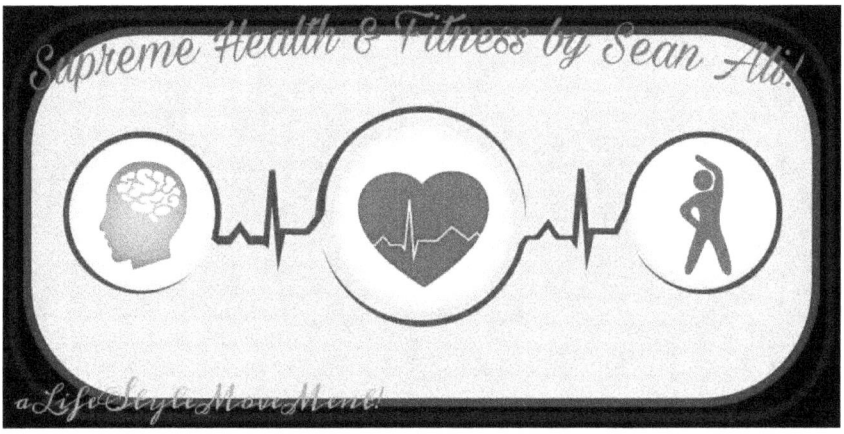

Achieving and Maintaining Supreme Health and Fitness by increasing the level of Knowledge and Science of LIFE!!!

Science Of Life Series......Volume One

OxyGen... The Breath Of Life In Atomic Form!

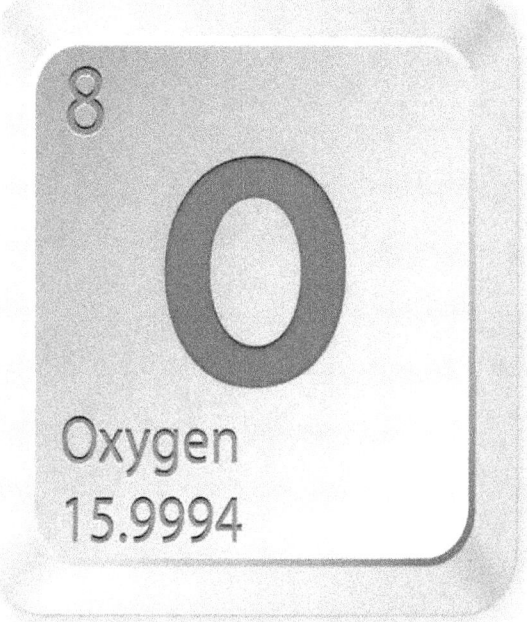

Atomic Form of the Breath Of LIFE!!

Supreme Health & Fitness!

Science Of Life Series... Vol 1

OxyGen ... The Breath Of Life In Atomic Form!

Table of Contents

*****

- Introduction ... . Page 10
- Chapter 1 .... Breath Of LIFE ... . Page 16
- Chapter 2 .... Everything is ATOMS ... . Page 22
- Chapter 3 .... Ozone, Air and Oxygen ... . Page 38
- Chapter 4 .... Respiratory System ... . Page 50
- Chapter 5 .... How Our Lungs Work ... . Page 60
- Chapter 6 .... Pulmonary Ventilation ... . Page 66
- Chapter 7 .... Oxygen, Blood and Hemoglobin ... . Page 76
- Chapter 8 .... Diaphragm ... . Page 80
- Chapter 9 .... Nasal Inhalation vs. Mouth ... . Page 86
- Chapter 10 .... Nasal Exhalation vs. Mouth ... . Page 98
- Chapter 11 .... OxyGen & Our Brain ... . Page 104
- Chapter 12 .... Oxidation and Oxidative Stress ... . Page 110
- Chapter 13 .... Respiration and Cellular Respiration ... . Page 116

OxyGen ... The Breath Of Life In Atomic Form!

- Chapter 14......Oxygen - Hypoxia, Free-Radicals & Cancer ... . Page 122
- Chapter 15......Oxygen and Anti-Oxidants ... . Page 128
- Chapter 16......Oxygen and Healing ... . Page 132
- Chapter 17......Conscious Breathing ... . Page 140
- Supreme Health & Fitness Heart Rate Test ... . Page 148
- Benefits Of Cardiovascular Exercise ... . Page 152
- Supreme Health & Fitness Fitness Walk Test ... . Page 158
- Supreme Health & Fitness 1.5 Mile Walk/Run Test ... . Page 160
- Supreme Health & Fitness Step Test ... . Page 162
- Supreme Health & Fitness Training Log ... . Page 164
- References and Resources ... . Page 166
- Publications by Supreme Health & Fitness ...

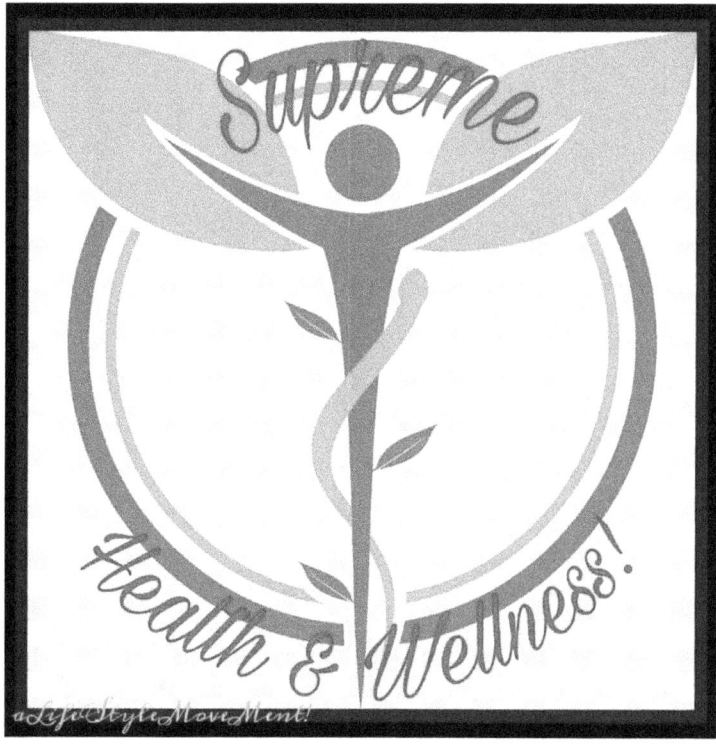

OxyGen ... The Breath Of Life In Atomic Form!

Introduction

*****

I Give ALL Praise and Honor to THE CREATOR and In the Name of GOD do I Humbly present this work ...

PEACE and BLESSINGS!

This small work represents the 1st Volume of my Science Of Life Series. In this Series we Scientifically exmine the Human Life, HOW it is Created to Funtion, WHAT it is made of, the proper Energy needed, and the BEST ways to Successfully perform our Life Functions.

    The purpose of this book is to Illustrate the Importance of Oxygen and to Offer that Oxygen IS The Breath Of LIFE in Atomic Form !

    We consider/measure the Basis of LIFE and Death on the criteria of the state of IF someone is Breathing or NOT. Breathing indicates LIFE. If someone is NOT Breathing we attempt Resuscitation to place the Breath of LIFE back into them. Depending on the conditions, the Breath of LIFE can Revive us after a state of Death (NOT Breathing).

    This is a direct Reflection of the Scriptural References to Our Creation. That we were Formed physically from the Dark Organic Matter of the Earth...however, were NOT considered ALIVE (Breathing), UNTIL we were Given the Breath Of LIFE (Resusetated – able to Breathe).

    I want to properly demonstrate the Law of Respiration (Inhaling and Exhaling) an that the Effects of Functioning in accordance - IS the Foundation for Successfully Achieving Abundant LIFE.

    I am HUMBLY attempting to draw the Connection between Breathing as Created vs. Breathing incorrectly and its direct correlation to ALL Sicknesses, Diseases and Pre-Mature Deaths that we currently Suffer from.

OxyGen ... The Breath Of Life In Atomic Form!

Particularly since it's reported that between the Ages 3-5, 96% of Us are BREATHING WRONG...which is the Direct CAUSE – with the Cancers and all other dis-eases being the Direct EFFECT.

The very foundation of our Physical Body is based on the Proper Functioning of Aerobic Cellular Respiration, of which OXYGEN (The Breath of LIFE) is The KEY Ingredient.

The Breath Of LIFE in the Atomic form of Oxygen, is the catalyst that allows Us to Manifest the Natural GOD POWER of Us. THE ABILITY TO SAY BE AND IT WILL (Our Thoughts/Will INFLUENCE the Shape of Atoms) BE !!!

It was the Search for an Understanding of myself that led me to concentrating my Focus (Thinking-Sight) to the Constant Realization that EVERYTHING is Simply ATOMS.

Building the Understanding, that in-order for me to Fully Understand myself, I had to Fully Understand the ATOM. That to Completely Understand and Manifest the POWER of myself, I had to Completely Understand the POWER of the ATOM.

We are SIMPLY ATOMS...so the LAWS that Govern the ATOM are the SAME that Govern Us.

So, the Natural Conclusion is that to Fully Understand and Govern myself, I had to Fully Understand the Laws that Govern the ATOM. Which is completely different then understanding and Manifesting Power, because many of Us Do so un-knowingly on a daily basis – we Mis-Understandingly Manifest Power. And it is in these conditions of 'unknowingly' and 'Lack of Understanding' that the Power Manifested makes CHAOS & CONFUSION.

Doing the Research and Gaining the Knowledge and Understanding of the ATOM and the Laws that govern it, LED ME TO THE 1st ATOM and GOD.

Scientific FACTS dictate that this 1st ATOMIC Particle (Foundation of LIFE) was dormant (Motionless) and that ONLY a HIGH ENERGY Could or Can MOVE an ATOMIC Particle = Beginning LIFE. The HIGHEST ENERGY IS GOD !

OxyGen … The Breath Of Life In Atomic Form!

The Standard Enthalpy of Formation for an Element in its Standard State is ZERO. Which means that Elements in their Standard State are NOT Formed, they JUST ARE - without Motion.

So, it was the THOUGHT OF THE CREATOR that Manifested into the Electro-Magnetic Charge that put that ATOMIC PARTICLE INTO MOTION = Start of LIFE and the LAWS that Govern the ATOM.

Thoughts Can and ARE Measured in/by Electrical Terms and Definition. Thoughts are Electro-Magnetic Energy that can SHAPE and ALTER the Laws that Govern the ATOM, the SAME fashion as the CREATOR did that Put that 1st ATOMIC Particle into MOTION.

This means an Unlimited and Un-Equal Potential POWER Of and In Us – Created in the Image and Likeness of GOD (Genesis 1:26)………IF WE OBEY THE LAWS OF THE CREATOR !!!!!

Since, we are ATOMS, I had to do further Research on How to Access the POWER of the ATOM and How to Connect the Physical Power that comes with the ATOM to the Mental-

Spiritual Power that comes with Psalms 82-6, 'You are all Gods, Children of the Most High' !

EVERYTHING IS ATOMS!!!

The Root Foundation of All LIFE is the ATOM, which everything – including Us is comprised of. So, it is quite Natural that the Breath Of LIFE also be found Manifested In Atomic Form !

The Purpose of this book is to Focus on and Address the Requirements of BREATHING on the ATOMIC Level and the resulting Atomic Power that's associated.

-We will Focus on and Discuss the Difference between AIR and OXYGEN.

-We will Focus on and Discuss the Importance of BREATHING as Created. -We will Focus on and Discuss the Effects of the BREATH of LIFE has on the Entire Body.

OxyGen ... The Breath Of Life In Atomic Form!

-We will Focus on and Discuss the 'CAUSE and EFFECTS' Law that is manifested from Breathing as Created and Breathing Other-than-Created.

-We will Focus on and Discuss the POWER of BREATHING.

-We will Focus on and Discuss How To Breathe To LIVE !

     We all Learn in the SAME fashion = REPITITION !! So, there may be Information REPEATED....this is done to reinforce the IMORTANCE of our Subject. + ``I want to Present my Scientific Knowledge and understanding in the Shortest and most Digestible form as possible.

I Pray that GOD is Pleased with my HUMBLE Endeavor..

PEACE and BLESSINGS !!

Your Brother,

Sean Ali

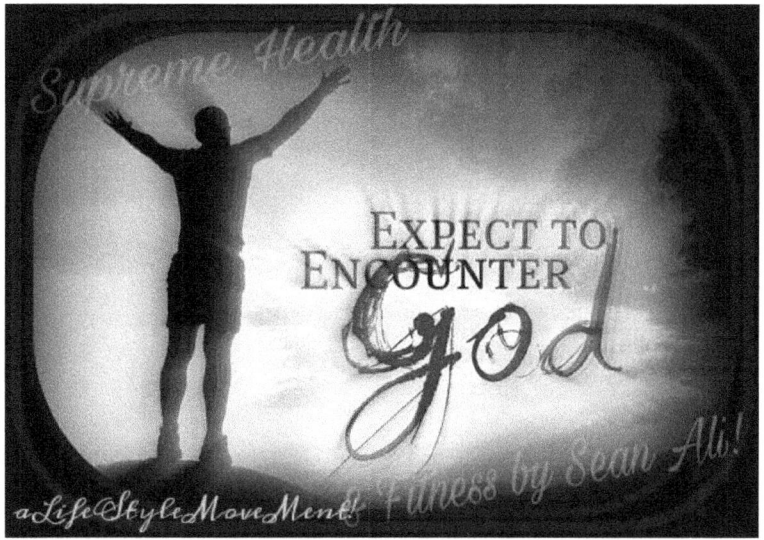

Chapter One ..... 'The Breath Of LIFE'

*

HOLY QUR'AN 32:9 – "Then HE proportioned him and BREATHED Into him from HIS Soul and made for you Hearing and Vision and Hearts; little are you Grateful."

****

GENESIS 2:7 – "Then The LORD GOD formed a Man from the Dust of the Ground and BREATHED Into his NOSTRILS The BREATH OF LIFE, and the Man became a LIVING BEING."

****

There are 3 Functions of *LIFE* that we MUST perform, as *Created*, in order to Successfully Build and Manifest the Highest Quality of Humanity = Being the Image & Likeness of GOD !

These 3 LIFE Functions are : <u>BREATHING</u> * <u>DRINKING</u> * <u>EATING</u> !

We can survive 1-3 weeks without Food. We can survive 3-6 days without Water.

WE CANNOT SURVIVE ANY LIMIT OF TIME WITHOUT BREATHIING !!!

We <u>CANNOT</u> go 1 Minute without Breathing Properly - without doing almost Irreparable Damage to the Cells/Tissue that comprises the Brain.

Within 3-6 Minutes, Brain/Mental Death and Irreversible Brain Damages are occurring.

So, out of the 3 Functions necessary for/to our LIFE.... BREATHING is the One Function that we <u>MUST</u> strive to Perform perfectly as Created.

OxyGen ... The Breath Of Life In Atomic Form!

The 1st LIFE Function that we Learn to Perform when we emerge from the Womb and into Existence is BREATHING......Which is a direct Representation of *The CREATOR* - Breathing the BREATH OF LIFE into the 1st Man. Making the Atomic Structure of Man LIVING !

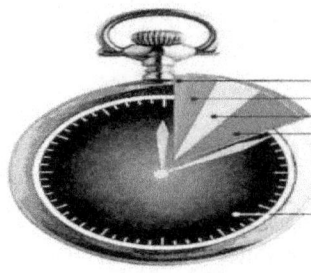

TIME IS CRITICAL!
0 to 1 minute: cardiac irritability
0 to 4 minutes: brain damage not likely
4 to 6 minutes: brain damage possible
6 to 10 minutes: brain damage very likely

More than 10 minutes: irreversible brain damage

The 1st Function that we Learn to Perform 'Other-than-Created' is BREATHING......And by the Ages 3-5, it is documented that 97% of us are BREATHING WRONG = MOUTH/CHEST Breathing.

The Activation and Development of the Foundation of All LIFE is Based-on/Dependent-upon the BREATH OF LIFE !

Being ALIVE is synonymous with the ACT of Breathing. When checking to see if someone is Alive – you check to see if they are Breathing.

A Heart-beat/Pulse and Brain Activity are by-products of the Act of Breathing.

Every Heart-beat first sends Blood to the LUNGS (Pulmonary Circuit) to become Oxygenated/Alive – BEFORE being dispersed thru the Body (Systemic Circuit), to Oxygenate/Activate the Brain and Body.

When someone is no longer Alive (not Breathing/no Heart-Beat), we Use OXYGEN in an attempt to Revive them. It is the Energy in/of the Breath Of LIFE in the Atomic form of Oxygen that is the KEY ingredient to LIFE

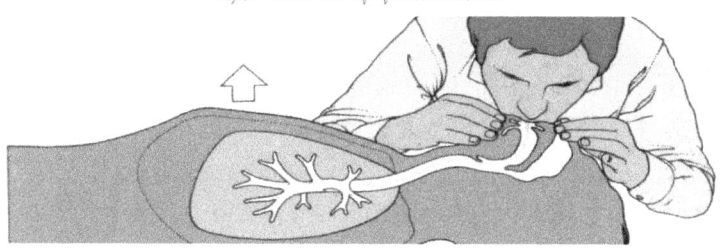

Cardiopulmonary (Mouth-to-Mouth) Resuscitation

Just as it was when The CREATOR used The Breath Of LIFE to START the LIFE/Heart of the 1st Man – we use that Breath Of LIFE in the form of Oxygen - to Resuscitate = Start the LIFE/Heart - to Revive a Dead person

The Breath Of LIFE – in the Atomic Form of Oxygen, provides the necessary Energy that Begins, Maintains and Increases the Rate of Rotation of our ATOMS = Giving/Bringing the Dead to LIFE !!

****

Hosea 4:6, *'My people are destroyed for LACK of Knowledge. Because you have rejected Knowledge, I will also reject you, that you shall be no priest to me. Since you have forgot the LAW of your GOD, I will also forget your children.'*

****

The Knowledge Of GOD is the Foundation of ALL Knowledge. We are Rooted IN GOD, so to be DESTROYED for a LACK of Knowledge – means that THAT Lack of Knowledge is ROOTED IN the Knowledge Of GOD !

The Knowledge Of Self has to take us to the ATOM (what we are Made of). The Knowledge of the ATOM reveals the WILL – Force and Power of GOD, that began the Rotation of the 1st Dormant Atomic Particle = the Beginning of LIFE.

So, the Knowledge Of GOD and the Knowledge Of Self are the Same. This is the Lack of Knowledge that is causing our Destruction.

The Knowledge of GOD is the Equivalent to the Breath Of LIFE for our Mental/Spiritual Bodies. The Knowledge Of GOD is the Electro-Magnetic Charge that is the Foundation for ALL Energies of LIFE.

Just as the Breath Of LIFE activated Man into Being a LIVING Soul and the Image and Likeness of GOD, the Knowledge Of GOD gives us the Qualifications to Manifest and Utilize the our God Force and Power.

The WILL Of GOD is Directly Expressed and Manifested IN the Laws that Govern LIFE…..So, to understand the Laws of LIFE is to Understand GOD.

So, the LACK of Knowledge that '*My People are destroyed from*' also encompasses the

Knowledge of the Laws …..Which is WHY 85% of the Population has the equivalent of NO LIFE !

Obedience to GOD is Manifested in and thru our Abilities to OBEY HIS Laws…….Wherein these Laws (particularly, Respiration) are adhered to = Life ABUNDANTLY !!

Disobedience = Destruction!!

OBEDIENCE = LIFE!!

There is NO mystery god… The Laws of the CREATOR include - '*CAUSE & EFFECT*'. The Science of HOW '**CAUSE & EFFECT**' functions, successfully eliminates ANY and ALL notions of any mystery god.

The **CAUSE** of Lack Of Knowledge to/of the Law of RESPIRATION = the **EFFECT** of Sicknesses, Illnesses, Dis-eases & Pre-Mature DEATH !

The **CAUSE** of BREATHING as Created = the **EFFECT** of Successfully Building and Maintaining Supreme Health and Fitness = *LIFE ABUNDANTLY* !

OxyGen ... The Breath Of Life In Atomic Form!

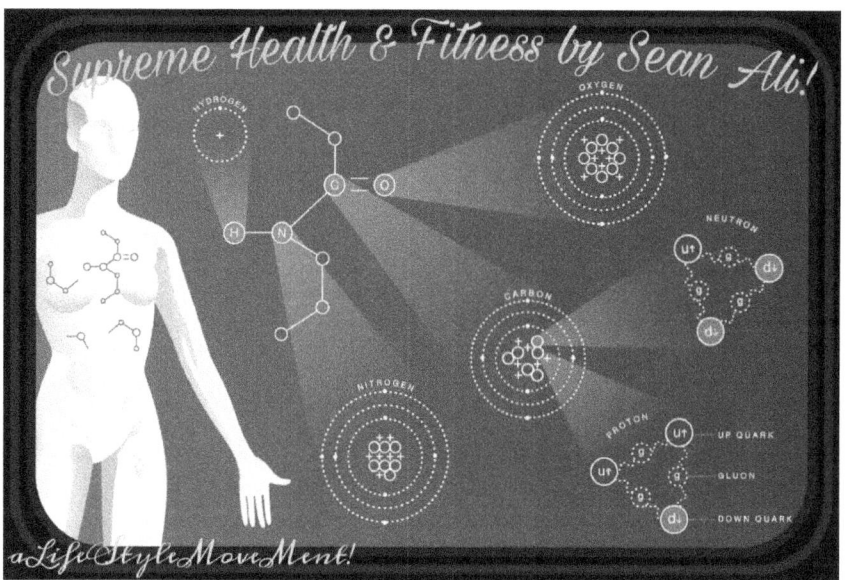

Oxygen ... The Breath Of Life In Atomic Form!

Chapter 2 ..... Everything Is ATOMS !!

******

There are a 92 Natural Atoms. These 92 Natural Atoms are the ingredients that make everything in LIFE, on Earth and in the Universe.

Atoms (with the Exception of Hydrogen, which has no Neutron) are Comprised of an EQUAL Number of Protons, Neutrons and Electrons.

The Protons and Neutrons are comprised of various Sub-Atomic Particles, or Fundamental Particles.

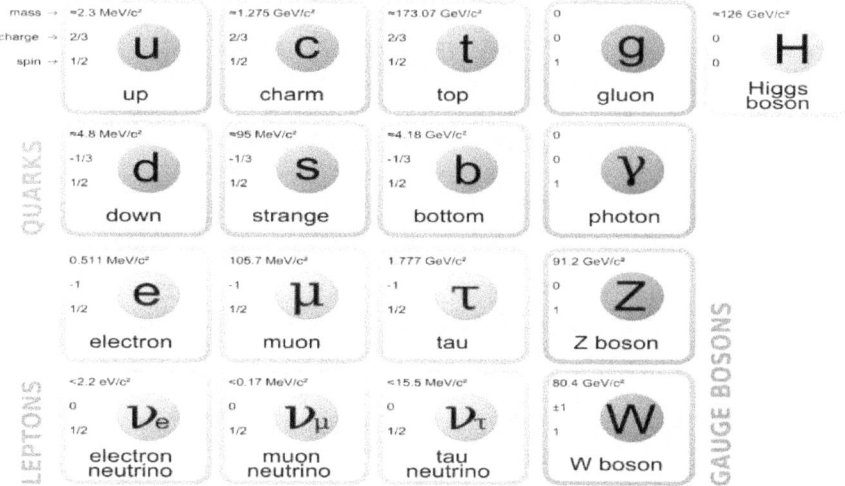

There are 2 Types of Sub-Atomic Particles – ELEMENTARY and COMPOSITE.

Elementary Particles are thought to NOT be made-up of other Particles.

OxyGen ... The Breath Of Life In Atomic Form!

Protons and Neutrons are Composite Particles. They are combined States of 2 or more Elementary Particles.

A Proton is made up of 2 UP-QUARKS and 1 DOWN-QUARK.

Neutrons are made of 2 DOWN-QUARKS and 1 UP-QUARKS.

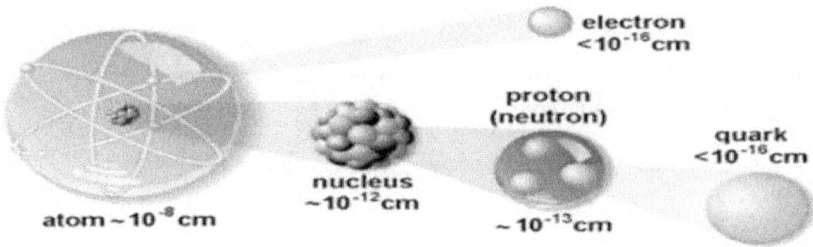

Other Composite Particles include – Hadrons, Baryons (Protons and Neutrons), Mesons (Pions and Haons) and Leptons.

All Composite Particles are Massive. Baryon means Heavy. Mesons means Inter-mediate and Leptons means Light-weight. Mass is expressed in terms of Energy. If a Particle has a Frame of Reference where it Lies At Rest, then it has a Positive Rest Mass and is referenced as Massive.

Any Particle with an Electrical Charge is considered Massive.

All Elementary Particles are considered MASS-LESS

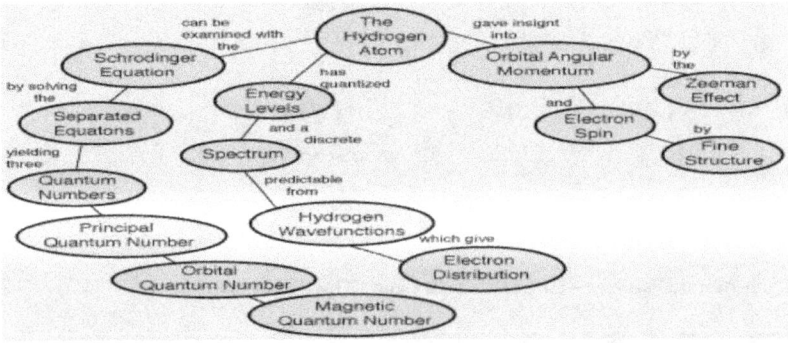

OxyGen ... The Breath Of Life In Atomic Form!

These Sub-Atomic Particles Attract each other and Bond to Form the Particles (Protons and Neutrons) – which forms ALL Atoms.

These Sub-Atomic Particles were put into Rotation by the STRONG Force (The WILL - Force and Power of THE CREATOR). They began to Build-up - Creating the 1st ATOM Hydrogen.

Electrons exist in layers referred to as Energy Layers or Shells.

As the Hydrogen Atom rotates and Attracts other Particles, it began Building-Up Neutrons and Electrons – Gaining Mass and Energy, while building up to eventually become another Element.

Hydrogen collected Particles, Building-Up to Helium.

At the Foundation of EVERY Atom is Hydrogen.

OxyGen ... The Breath Of Life In Atomic Form!

To KNOW the ATOM is to KNOW SELF !!!

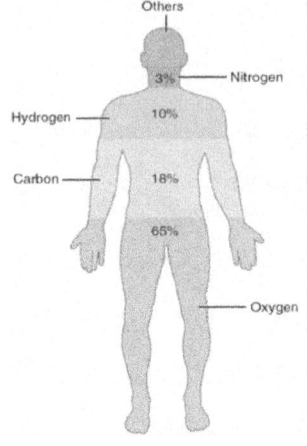

Element	Symbol	Percentage in Body
Oxygen	O	65.0
Carbon	C	18.5
Hydrogen	H	9.5
Nitrogen	N	3.2
Calcium	Ca	1.5
Phosphorus	P	1.0
Potassium	K	0.4
Sulfur	S	0.3
Sodium	Na	0.2
Chlorine	Cl	0.2
Magnesium	Mg	0.1
Trace elements include boron (B), chromium (Cr), cobalt (Co), copper (Cu), fluorine (F), iodine (I), iron (Fe), manganese (Mn), molybdenum (Mo), selenium (Se), silicon (Si), tin (Sn), vanadium (V), and zinc (Zn).		less than 1.0

These are the Atomic Elements that Create Us

*The Breath Of LIFE (OXYGEN) is the Most Abundant ATOMIC Element.

*CARBON (the Dark Organic Material Used to Fashion the Physical) is the 2nd Most.

*HYDROGEN (1st ATOM and Foundation of Life) is 3rd and is a BINDING Element, especially thru Hydrogen Bonds.

*NITROGEN is 4th and very Important in the Functions of LIFE. Nitrogen helps with Cellular Re-Generation,

Prevention of Dis-Eases, Proper functioning of Reproductive System and Proper operations of our Hearts/Circulatory System.

*CALCIUM is our 5th abundant and major element in the mineralization of our Skeletal (Bone, Teeth) structure as well being essential for Cell physiology of all living Organisms.

*PHOSPHORUS is the last major Element that id vital to the process of Metabolism in Self. Phosphorus is also LIGHT...THE LIGHT (which is Our ATOMIC make-up) that THE CREATOR used from With-In HIMSELF to Manifest the LIGHT Out-Side HIMSELF.

OxyGen ... The Breath Of Life In Atomic Form!

The Phosphorus in Our ATOMIC make-up helps to capture and convert the Energy of SUN into Chemical compounds used for Cellular Growth and Development.

The Configuration of Electrons determines the way in which Atoms react with each other – referred to as its Chemical Prosperities. These Chemical Properties form the Basis for the Bonding of Atoms, which directly effects the formation/out-come of the completed Atomic Composition. These Chemical Properties form our DNA, which is the Foundation for our Creation.

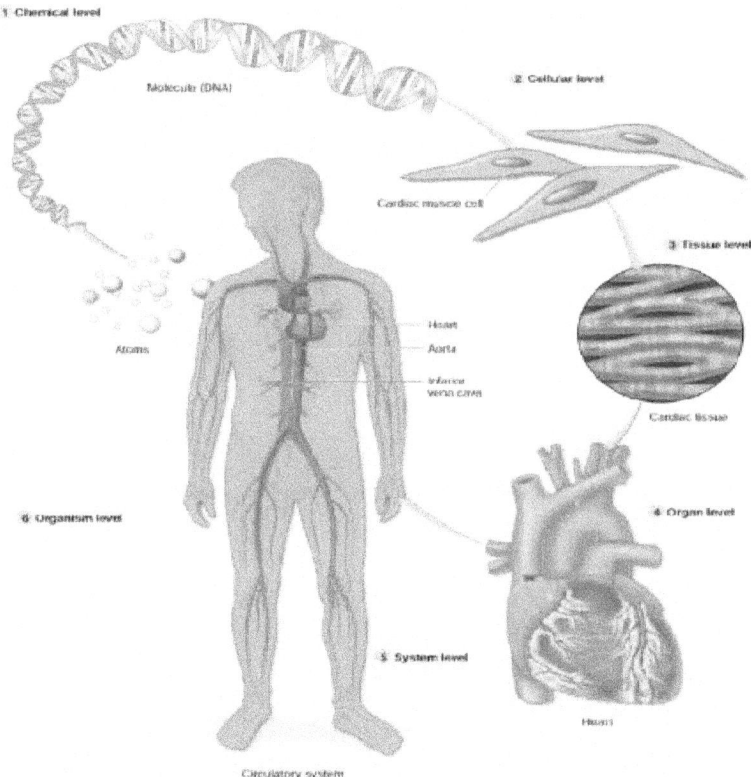

Atoms Gain, Lose or Share Electrons when they Bond to form Molecules.

The Configurations formed from the Bonding are the Determining Factor to what type of Atomic Structure is being Created.

Electrons exist in layers referred to as Energy Layers or Shells.

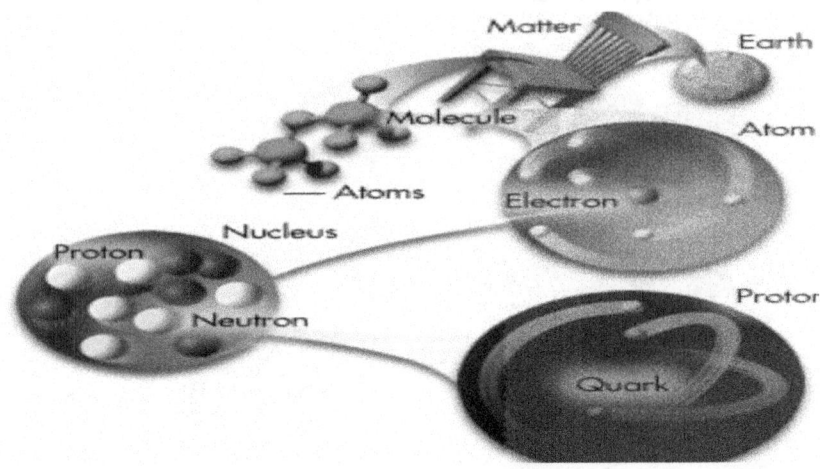

*Chemistry is the Study of HOW the Sharing of Electrons Binds Atoms and Causes them React.

*Nuclear Physics is the Study of HOW Protons and Neutrons Arrange themselves in Nuclei.

*Particle Physics (also known as Quantum Physics) is the Study of Sub-Atomic Particles, Atoms and Molecules and their Structure and Inter-Actions.

*High Energy Physics is the Study of the HIGH ENERGY that is Required to Create Sub-Atomic Particles.

This HIGH ENERGY is the Thought (WILL, FORCE and POWER) of THE CREATOR that

OxyGen ... The Breath Of Life In Atomic Form!

Manifested in Electro-Magnetic Energy which MOVED the Sub-Atomic Particles = The START OF LIFE !

EVERYTHING IS ATOMS !!

To Understand the ATOM is to Understand SELF – for Self is but an ATOM - Multiplied and Built-Up upon itself.

EVERYTHING IS ATOMS !!

To Understand ATOMIC Power is to Understand Human Power !

EVERYTHING IS ATOMS !!

To Understand Breathing on the ATOMIC Level is Key to Obtaining the Foundation to the Fountain of YOUTH !!

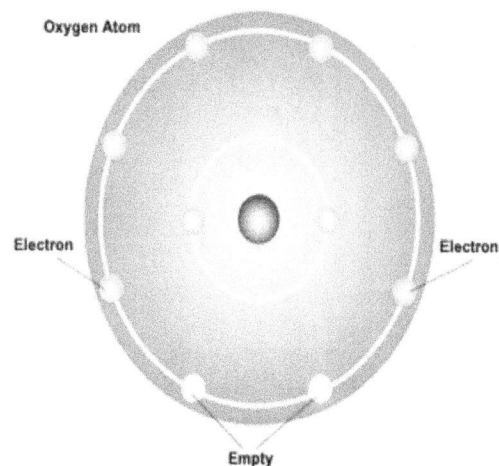

A Single Oxygen Atom

The Outer Shell can hold up to 8 Electrons. The 2 available positions are for Bonding with another Atom to form an Element.

OxyGen ... The Breath Of Life In Atomic Form!

Atomic Knowledge Of Self

We Humans, as well as the rest of the Living, are made of multiple Chemicals, but of them all there are Four Elements that predominate: **Oxygen**, **Carbon**, **Hydrogen**, and **Nitrogen**. For every **1,000 Atoms** in our bodies, approximately **630** are **Hydrogen**, **255** are **Oxygen**, **95** are **Carbon**, and **15** are **Nitrogen**. We also contain small quantities of **Calcium**, **Phosphorus** and **Sulfur**, **Sodium**, **Chlorine**, and **Magnesium**.

Although trace elements are less abundant in the body, some of them are necessary for Life, such as **Iron**, **Iodine**, and **Selenium**. Most of these trace elements are for sale at your local pharmacy, next to the multivitamins. However, they are needed in extremely small doses—minute traces, in fact—so taking **ANY** supplemental minerals will enhance bodily performance **ONLY** if your diet lacks them to begin with.

Atomic Structure Is the Foundation of Life

Elements are made of **Atoms**, and Atoms are mostly **empty space**. Atoms include a central **Nucleus** with an ill-defined **space** surrounding it. A cloud of Electrons resides in this space, **orbiting** the Nucleus.

The **Electrons** stay in orbit through **Electrical attraction** to the **Positive Protons** of the Nucleus. Atoms are the basis for the Chemical world, and each Atom is the smallest possible sample of a particular Element.

Most Atoms can react with other Elements to form Compounds and Molecules.

OxyGen ... The Breath Of Life In Atomic Form!

Atoms are composed of **Neutrons**, **Protons**, and **Electrons**. **Neutrons** and **Protons** are always in the **Nucleus**, and the **Electrons** move rapidly around the **Nucleus**. Elements are defined by the **number** of **Protons**; all **Atoms** of a particular element have the **same number** of **Protons**. **Protons** and **Neutrons** each have a mass of approximately **One Dalton**; **Electrons** are far less massive.

Neutron: The neutral particle in the Atomic Nucleus.

Proton: The positive particle in the Atomic Nucleus.

Electron: The negative particle in an Atom, found in orbitals surrounding the Nucleus.

Mass: The amount of "substance" in an object. ("Weight" is the mass under a particular amount of Gravity.)

Isotopes: Elements with the same number of Protons but different numbers of Neutrons, resulting in different Atomic Masses.

Atomic Number: The number of Protons in the Nucleus of an Atom.

Atomic Mass: The total weight of Neutrons and Protons of an Atom; different Isotopes have different Atomic Masses.

Radioactive: decay, spontaneous disintegration of a Radioactive substance into another element through Nuclear Division and the release of Energy.

Ion: A charged Atom

Many elements have **Isotopes**, with the same number of **Protons** but a different number of Neutrons. All Isotopes of a particular element are chemically identical but have different masses, owing to the change in neutrons. The **number** of **Neutrons equals** the **Atomic Mass minus** the **Atomic Number**. The **Atomic Mass** recorded in the **Periodic Table** is an average mass for the Element.

Adding or subtracting **Protons** from a Nucleus creates a new element. New elements form inside stars, nuclear reactors, and nuclear bombs. They also form through Radioactive Decay.

When these unstable **Isotopes break apart**, they **release Energy** and **form less massive Atoms**, which may break again into other Elements.

OxyGen ... The Breath Of Life In Atomic Form!

The emitted Energy can be helpful or harmful.

The number of Electrons always equals the number of Protons in a neutral (uncharged) Atom. Protons have a positive charge and a mass, whereas Electrons carry a negative charge but no appreciable mass. The Electromagnetic Attraction between Protons and Electrons prevents the Electrons from leaving the Atom.

The Positive–Negative attraction between Proton and Electron resembles the north–south attraction between refrigerator magnets and steel refrigerator doors.

The outermost Energy level of Electrons, or Valence shell, is most important in chemistry and biology because that is where Atoms Bond. The Roman numeral above each column in the Periodic Table indicates the number of Valence Electrons of all the Atoms in that column.

Ions and Chemical Bonds are important with-in our bodies

In chemistry, the Periodic Table organizes all Elements in a logical pattern, according to Atomic Number. As you now know, the Atomic Number is the number of Protons in the Nucleus.

The table also reveals an Element's reactivity - its ability to Bond with other Elements, as reflected in the Valence Electrons.

Elements in a particular column have the same number of Valence Electrons, and thus similar reactive properties. If we are familiar with any element in a column, we can predict the reactivity of other Elements in that column.

IIIA	IVA	VA	VIA	VIIA
5 Boron **B** 10.811	6 Carbon **C** 12.011	7 Nitrogen **N** 14.007	8 Oxygen **O** 15.999	9 Fluorine **F** 18.998
13 Aluminum **Al** 26.9815	14 Silicon **Si** 28.086	15 Phosphorus **P** 30.974	16 Sulfur **S** 32.066	17 Chlorine **Cl** 35.453

The Periodic Table lists each Element by a standard one- or two-letter abbreviations.

Chemistry - Science of Bonding

Chemistry is a science of Bonds being created and Bonds being broken. Bonds between Atoms determine how Chemical Compounds form, fall apart, and re-form.

For an example, when we metabolize sugar, we are essentially combining its Carbon and Hydrogen Atoms with Oxygen, forming Carbon Dioxide and Water. These reactions produce Heat and Energy that our body uses for just about every Life function and purpose. If we don't use sugar and related compounds immediately, some of them are converted to Fat—larger Molecules that store even more Energy in their Chemical Bonds.

Life is created of Atoms, but Atoms are only the building-blocks of Molecules and chemical compounds. A Molecule is a chemical unit formed from two or more Atoms. H2, for example, is a Molecule of Hydrogen.

A Compound is a Molecule with unlike Atoms: CO2, Carbon Dioxide, is both a Molecule and a Compound. The chemical properties of a Compound have little or nothing to do with the properties that make-up the Atoms. Sodium, for example, is a soft metal that burns when exposed to Air. Chlorine is a toxic gas at room temperature, but Sodium Chloride is table salt. Of course, the Atoms individually are, not alive. Once they combine and become part of us and our environment, however, they become the ingredients of Life.

Chemical bonds are a matter of Electrons. Atoms without a "filled" Valence Shell adhere to one another by sharing or moving Electrons. Atoms can bond in three common ways, ranging in strength from the strong Ionic Bonds of Salts and the equally strong Shared Bonds of Organic Molecules to the weak Hydrogen Bonds that hold DNA Molecules together:

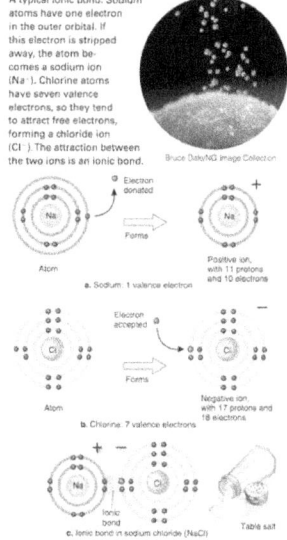

A typical ionic bond: Sodium atoms have one electron in the outer orbital. If this electron is stripped away, the atom becomes a sodium ion (Na⁻). Chlorine atoms have seven valence electrons, so they tend to attract free electrons, forming a chloride ion (Cl⁻). The attraction between the two ions is an ionic bond. Bruce Dale/NG Image Collection

1. The Ionic Bond holds Ions in a Compound, based on the strong attraction between Positive and Negative Ions—something like the north–south attraction between a refrigerator magnet and refrigerator door discussed previously. The **interactions** between Sodium and Chlorine show a typical ionic bond (see Figure).

Many **Ions** in the human body, including Calcium (Ca2+), Sodium (Na+), Potassium (K+), Hydrogen (H+), Phosphate (PO43-), Bicarbonate (HCO3-), Chloride (Cl-), and Hydroxide (OH-), can form **Ionic Bonds**. All these Ions play significant roles in our ability to achieve **Homeostasis**.

In some people, too much Sodium can raise Blood Pressure. Too little Calcium causes soft, weak bones, as in rickets, and Potassium and Calcium imbalances can cause heart irregularities. The other Ions are vital to maintaining the blood's acid/base balance.

OxyGen ... The Breath Of Life In Atomic Form!

If Ion levels do not stay within normal range, Cellular functions can cease, leading to the death of Tissues, Organs, and even the Organism = Us.

2. Although Ions are common in the body, Covalent Bonds are actually more important to Living Tissue than are Ionic Bonds. In Covalent bonds, Atoms share Electrons; Electrons are not donated by one Atom and grabbed by another, as in an Ionic bond.

Covalent bonds commonly involve Carbon, Oxygen, Nitrogen, or Hydrogen, the elements predominant in our Life. In a Covalent bond, Atoms share Electrons so that each gets to complete its Valence Shell.

Two Atoms share one pair of Electrons in a Single Covalent Bond, as occurs in a Hydrogen Molecule. Single Covalent Bonds are shown in chemical diagrams as one line: H- H.

In a Double Covalent Bond, 2 pairs of Electrons are shared. For example, two Oxygen Atoms form an Oxygen Molecule (O2) by sharing 4 electrons. Each Oxygen

Because of the stronger pull the oxygen atom exerts on the shared electrons, they spend more time encircling the oxygen nucleus. This difference in electronegativity results in a polar molecule. The oxygen end is slightly negative, while the hydrogen atoms carry a partially positive charge.

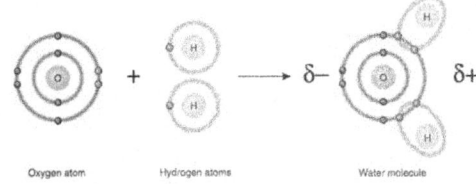

Oxygen atom   Hydrogen atoms   Water molecule

Atom has 6 Electrons in its Valence shell; with the addition of two more electrons, it gets that stable shell of 8 electrons. **Double Covalent Bonds** are shown in chemical diagrams with a double line: O= O.

In a **Triple Covalent Bond**, 3 pairs of Electrons are shared. This is the way that two Atoms of Nitrogen form a Nitrogen Molecule (N2). Nitrogen has 5 Electrons in its Valence Shell; by sharing 6 Electrons between the two, each can add 3 Electrons, making 8 in the Valence Shell. Triple Covalent Bonds are shown as a triple line: N N.

3. The Hydrogen Bond is weak but vital to Biology. When a Hydrogen Atom is part of a Polar Covalent Bond, the Hydrogen end of the Molecule tends to be more positive, leaving the other end more negative. The result is a Molecule with a charge gradient along its length.

The slight positive charge of the Hydrogen Atom can form weak attractive bonds with adjacent, slightly negative atoms in other Compounds. Although the Hydrogen Bond is too weak to bond Atoms in the same way as Covalent or Ionic bonds, it does cause attractions between nearby Molecules. Hydrogen Bonds join the two strands of DNA (our Genetic material) in the Nucleus of our Cells. They also help shape Proteins, the building blocks of Living bodies.

OxyGen ... The Breath Of Life In Atomic Form!

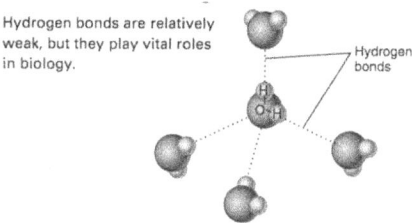

Hydrogen bonds are relatively weak, but they play vital roles in biology.

Hydrogen Bonds occur between Water Molecules because the Electrons of the Covalent bond between Hydrogen and Oxygen preferentially circle the Oxygen Nucleus. With more negative charges around the Oxygen, the result is a partially negative Oxygen Atom and a partially positive Hydrogen Atom.

The partially negative Oxygen in one Molecule is attracted to the partially positive Hydrogen Atoms of another Molecule.

Bonds Do More Than Hold Atoms Together in Molecules

One of the basic concepts in our human biology is the storage and transfer of Energy. Biological organisms - Us included - use Energy at a tremendous rate to carry out the processes of our Life (not including any extra exertion as with exercising). For us, this Energy is obtained from the foods we eat. More specifically, this Energy is obtained from the Bonds that hold together the Atoms in the foods that we eat. This **storage** and **transfer** of Energy is a simple concept, but it is paramount to much that occurs in the body.

Energy Is Stored in All Types of Chemical Bonds

It takes Energy to hold Atoms together in Molecules. No matter which type of Bond is employed - hydrogen, covalent, or ionic - Energy within that specific Bond is holding the Atoms together. Large complex Molecules will not spontaneously form from Atoms if Energy is not added to the Reaction.

For example, Carbon Atoms do not come together to form Glucose on their own. Plants and other photosynthesizing organisms collect Solar Energy and use that to connect Carbon Atoms and form Sugars. Solar Energy is harvested in specialized parts of the plant Cells and used to create Sugar by aiding in the formation of Carbon to carbon bonds.

The energy that was part of the Sun's output now resides in the bonds that hold the sugar molecule together.

OxyGen ... The Breath Of Life In Atomic Form!

Periodic Table and Elements

The Periodic Table lists the known chemical elements, which are considered the basic units of Matter. The Elements in the table are arranged left to right in rows in order of their Atomic Number, the number of Protons in the Nucleus.

Each horizontal row, numbered from 1 to 7, is a Period. All Elements in a given Period have the same number of electron shells as their period number. For example, an Atom of Hydrogen or Helium each has one Electron Shell, while an Atom of Potassium or Calcium each has four Electron Shells.

The Elements in each column, or group, share chemical properties. For example, the Elements in column IA are very chemically reactive, whereas the elements in column VIIIA have full Electron Shells and thus are chemically inert.

Scientists now recognize up to 118 different elements; of these, 92 occur naturally on Earth, and the rest (with the exception of element 117) **have been produced synthetically using particle accelerators**.

Twenty-six of the 92 naturally occurring Elements normally are present in your body. Of these, just **4 Elements** - **Oxygen** (O), **Carbon** (C), **Hydrogen** (H), and **Nitrogen** (N) (coded blue)—constitute about 96% of the body's Mass.

Eight others - **Calcium** (Ca), **Phosphorus** (P), **Potassium** (K), **Sulfur** (S), **Sodium** (Na), **Chlorine** (Cl), **Magnesium** (Mg), and **Iron** (Fe) (coded pink)—contribute **3.8%** of the **Body's Mass**.

An additional **14 Elements**, called **Trace Elements** because they are present in tiny amounts, account for the remaining **0.2%** of the **Body's Mass**.

The **Trace Elements** are **Aluminum**, **Boron**, **Chromium**, **Cobalt**, **Copper**, **Fluorine**, Iodine, **Manganese**, **Molybdenum**, Selenium, Silicon, Tin, **Vanadium**, and **Zinc** (coded yellow).

OxyGen ... The Breath Of Life In Atomic Form!

Periodic Table of the Elements

Percentage of body mass:
- 96% (4 elements)
- 3.8% (8 elements)
- 0.2% (14 elements)

Legend: 23 = Atomic number, V = Chemical symbol, 50.942 = Atomic mass (weight)

IA	IIA	IIIB	IVB	VB	VIB	VIIB	VIIIB	VIIIB	VIIIB	IB	IIB	IIIA	IVA	VA	VIA	VIIA	VIIIA
1 H 1.0079																	2 He 4.003
3 Li 6.941	4 Be 9.012											5 B 10.811	6 C 12.011	7 N 14.007	8 O 15.999	9 F 18.998	10 Ne 20.180
11 Na 22.989	12 Mg 24.305											13 Al 26.9815	14 Si 28.086	15 P 30.974	16 S 32.066	17 Cl 35.453	18 Ar 39.948
19 K 39.098	20 Ca 40.08	21 Sc 44.956	22 Ti 47.87	23 V 50.942	24 Cr 51.996	25 Mn 54.938	26 Fe 55.845	27 Co 58.933	28 Ni 58.69	29 Cu 63.546	30 Zn 65.38	31 Ga 69.723	32 Ge 72.59	33 As 74.992	34 Se 78.96	35 Br 79.904	36 Kr 83.80
37 Rb 85.468	38 Sr 87.62	39 Y 88.905	40 Zr 91.22	41 Nb 92.906	42 Mo 95.94	43 Tc (99)	44 Ru 101.07	45 Rh 102.905	46 Pd 106.42	47 Ag 107.868	48 Cd 112.40	49 In 114.82	50 Sn 118.69	51 Sb 121.75	52 Te 127.60	53 I 126.904	54 Xe 131.30
55 Cs 132.905	56 Ba 137.33		72 Hf 178.49	73 Ta 180.948	74 W 183.85	75 Re 186.2	76 Os 190.2	77 Ir 192.22	78 Pt 195.08	79 Au 196.967	80 Hg 200.59	81 Tl 204.38	82 Pb 207.19	83 Bi 208.980	84 Po (209)	85 At (210)	86 Rn (222)
87 Fr (223)	88 Ra (226)		104 Rf (261)	105 Db (262)	106 Sg (263)	107 Bh (264)	108 Hs (269)	109 Mt (268)	110 Uun (281)	111 Uuu (272)	112 Uub (277)	113 Uut (284)	114 Uuq (289)	115 Uup (288)	116 Uuh (293)		118 Uuo (294)

57-71, Lanthanides

57 La 138.91	58 Ce 140.12	59 Pr 140.907	60 Nd 144.24	61 Pm 144.913	62 Sm 150.35	63 Eu 151.96	64 Gd 157.25	65 Tb 158.925	66 Dy 162.50	67 Ho 164.930	68 Er 167.26	69 Tm 168.934	70 Yb 173.04	71 Lu 174.97

89-103, Actinides

89 Ac (227)	90 Th 232.038	91 Pa (231)	92 U 238.03	93 Np (237)	94 Pu 244.064	95 Am (243)	96 Cm (247)	97 Bk (247)	98 Cf 242.058	99 Es (254)	100 Fm 257.095	101 Md 258.10	102 No 259.10	103 Lr 260.105

OxyGen ... The Breath Of Life In Atomic Form!

Chapter 3 ..... Ozone, Air & Oxygen

*****

Ozone, Air and **Oxygen** are sometimes thought of and used interchangeably, but they are **3** Separate **Elements**, formed from the **Atomic Element Oxygen.**

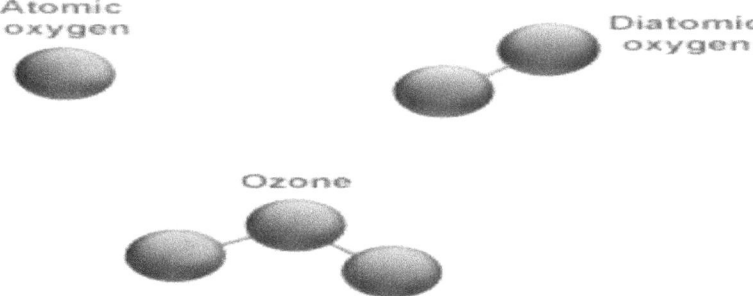

The differences arise in the types of **Reactions** on the **Oxygen Atoms** that occur to form each **Element**.

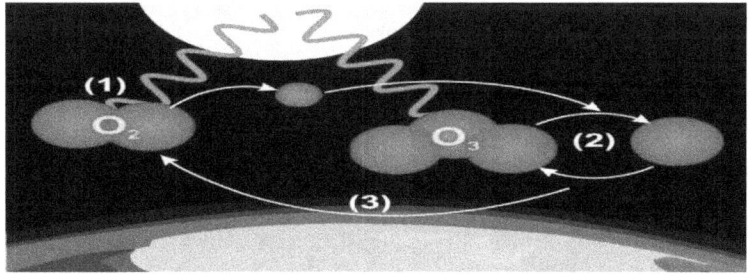

The **Breath Of LIFE** (in the **Atomic** form of **Oxygen**) isn't just responsible for **LIFE**, but in various formations - **Oxygen** is our **Protective Barrier** as our Planet travels on its Rotation around the **Sun**.

> The term **Ozone** refers to the **Natural Reaction** of the Sun (**Ultra-Violet rays**) breaking up the **Molecule** (**2 Oxygen Atoms Bonded**) of **Oxygen**. The **UV Rays** breaks the **Covalent Bonds** of the **Molecules** of **Oxygen**, creating Single **Atomic** Particles of **Oxygen**.

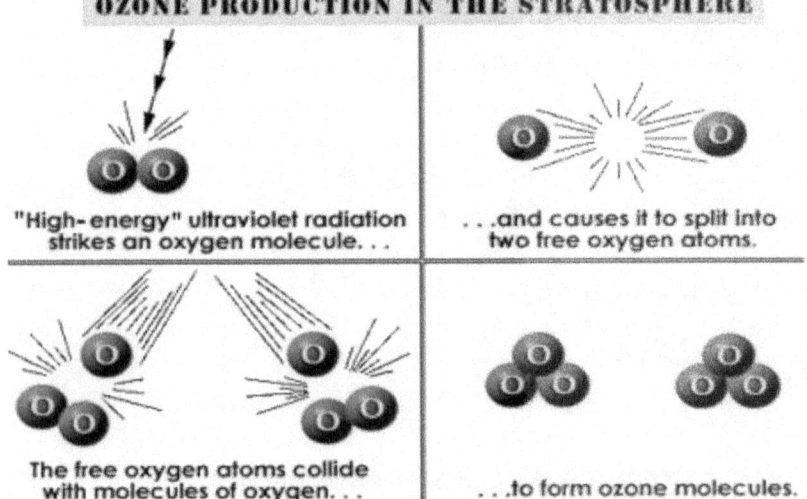

These individual **Atoms** of **Oxygen** collide with other **Molecules** of **Atoms** – causing the **Reaction** of the single **Atomic Oxygen** to **BOND** with the **Molecule** of **Oxygen** – forming **OZONE Molecule** (**3 Oxygen Atoms Bonded**).

The Formula for **Ozone** is **O3**.

Ozone Gas is an **Allotrope** – Form of the **Element Oxygen**.

The **Reaction** that creates **Ozone** occurs in the **Stratosphere**. In-turn, **Ozone** Protects **LIFE** on Earth from the most **Harmful** (**UV-B** Radiation) and **Destructive** (**UV-C** Radiation) SUN Rays.

90% Of the **Stratosphere** is **Ozone** (**O3**). Between the Distances of **15 - 50** KM from the **Earths Surface** constitutes the **Area** of the **Stratosphere**.

OxyGen ... The Breath Of Life In Atomic Form!

Ozone constitutes approximately **10%** of the make-up of the **Troposphere**. From the **Earths Surface** to **15 – 20** KM is the **Area** in **Distance** of the **Troposphere**. When **Ozone** exceeds **10%**, it **Damages** our **Respiratory Tissues**.

Ozone is an **In-Organic Molecule**. It has an **Odor** that's **Sharp** and similar to **Chlorine**.

> The term **Air** is used to refer to the **Earth's Atmosphere** as a whole.

What Is AIR?

- The layer of gases that surrounds the Earth is called the atmosphere.
  - The atmosphere holds in heat from the sun keeping the Earth's surface at a comfortable temperature.
  - The atmosphere protects living things from harmful rays given off by the sun.

Air forms the lower part of the **Atmosphere**. **Air** is a mixture that contains primarily **Oxygen – 21%** and **Nitrogen – 78%**, with other **Gases** of **Carbon Dioxide, Hydrogen, Helium, Argon** and **Neon** combining to make up the remainder **1%**.

The **Reaction** that creates **Air** takes place in the **Troposphere,** or as its commonly referred to as - **Atmosphere**.

At **Sea** Level, the **Ratio** of **21%** **Oxygen** & **78%** **Nitrogen** remains....Above **Sea** Level, **Air** becomes **Thinner** (**Oxygen** percentage **DECREASED**)......Below Sea Level, **Air** becomes **Thicker** (**Oxygen** percentage **Increased**).

Air Molecules

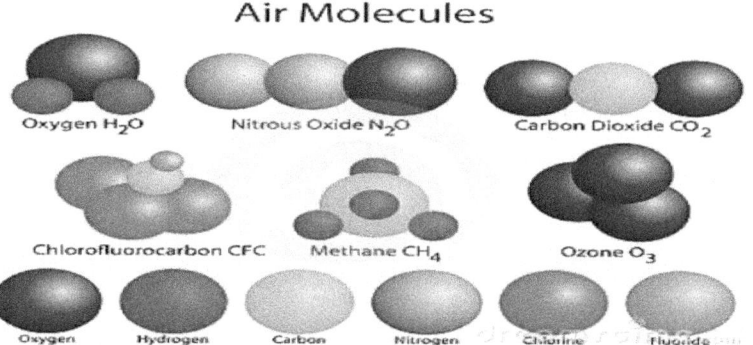

Oxygen H_2O — Nitrous Oxide N_2O — Carbon Dioxide CO_2
Chlorofluorocarbon CFC — Methane CH_4 — Ozone O_3
Oxygen — Hydrogen — Carbon — Nitrogen — Chlorine — Fluoride

OxyGen ... The Breath Of Life In Atomic Form!

All of the **Molecules** of **Air**, have **Weight** to them, individually and combined. The **Combined Weight** causes a **Pressure** of **10,000 KG Per Square Meter, DOWN** on our **Bodies**.

This means that the **Mass** of **Air** above the **0.1 Square Meter Cross-Section** of our **Bodies** is **1,000 KG** or **1 Tonnage**. We aren't **CRUSHED** by this enormous **Pressure** because the **Air Pressure** in our **Lungs**, **Ears** and **Stomachs**, maintain the **SAME** amount of **Pressure** as Outside. **EQUALIZING** and **Neutralizing** the **Pressure**, allowing us to constantly and continually **Move** at **Will**.

Yawning, Ears-Popping, Belching and Flatulence, are all examples of reactions from our **Bodies** attempting to **Equalize Pressure** when we have done something (ate, drank or used Mouth to Breathe) to throw-off that **Balance**.

Air contains a wide-variety of **Molecules**. Including : **Nitrous Oxide - N2O, Carbon Dioxide – CO2, Ozone – O3** and **Oxygen – O2** (as well as several others), that support all the various forms of **LIFE** on our **Planet**.

All these forms of **LIFE** are created with the adequate **Respiratory System,** necessary to Extract their specific **Molecule** from the many that comprise **Air**.

A **Breath** of Inhaled **Air** contains approximately **21%** **Oxygen Molecules**.

> The term **Oxygen** refers to the **Natural Non-Metallic Atomic Element**.

Oxygen is a **Pure Gaseous Element** with the **Atomic Weight** of **8 = 8 Protons, 8 Neutrons, 8 Electrons**.

Oxygen Gas is the **2nd** most common **Component** of **Earth's Biosphere = Air**, **Sea** and **Land**. It is approximately **20.8%** of the **Earth's Atmospheric VOLUME** and **23.1%** of the **Atmospheric MASS**. **Oxygen** is also approximately **49.5%** of the material that comprises the **Earth's Crust**.

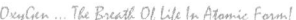

Oxygen ... The Breath Of Life In Atomic Form!

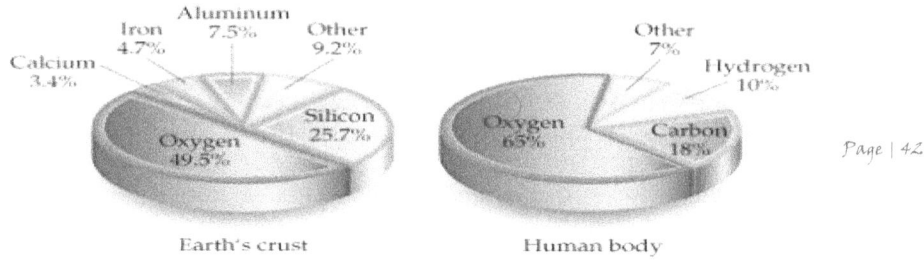

Earth's crust   Human body

Oxygen is Naturally constitutes approximately **65%** of the **Atomic** make-up of our **Bodies**.

So, when we **DON'T Breathe** as created, the **Natural Atomic Composition** of our **Physical** is thrown-off Balance and disrupted.

This makes us Other-than our **Natural Atomic Selves**.

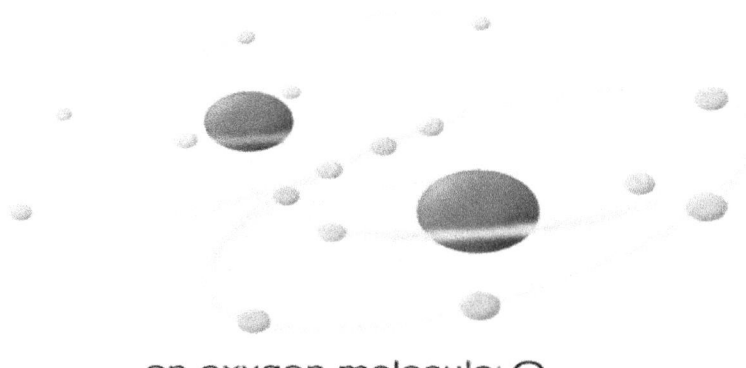

an oxygen molecule: O_2

The **Oxygen** we **Breathe** is comprised of **2 Oxygen Atoms Bonded** held thru a **DOUBLE COVALENT BOND**. The **Covalent Bond Energy of Oxygen is 119 Kcal/Mol**.

A **Double Covalent Bond** is when **Atoms** are **Bonded** by **2** pairs of their **Electrons**. This creates a **Stable Molecule**.

Oxygen is the Most abundant **Element** in the **Earths** crust (mainly in the forms of **Oxides, Silicates, Carbonates**), constituting approximately **49.2%** of the Crusts **MASS**.

OxyGen ... The Breath Of Life In Atomic Form!

Oxygen constitutes **88.8%** of the **Earth's Waters (Ocean's, Rivers, Lakes**) **Oxygen** comprises approximately **0.9%** of the **Sun's MASS**.

The average Level of **Oxygen** in our **Blood** should be approximately **96%**...any **Lower** results in **OXIDATION**, which negatively affects our **Cellular** Health, Growth and Development.

When we have a Level **LOWER** than **96%** = **Oxygen** Deficient, it creates the environment for **Free-Radicals** (Un-stable **Atoms**) to be formed/increased. A **LOW** Level of **Oxygen** can only by derived from **NOT Breathing** as created = **Mouth** and **Chest Breathing**.

Health that is affected by **LOW** Levels of **Oxygen** includes (but not limited to):

*****Brain Damage**. The **Brain** consumes **20%** Of the **Oxygen** inhaled. Lack-of/Low **Oxygen** creates a Weak/SLOW Processing (Thinking, Activation) **Brain**. Since the **Brain** REGULATES the Entire **Body** = A Weak/Slow Total **Body**.

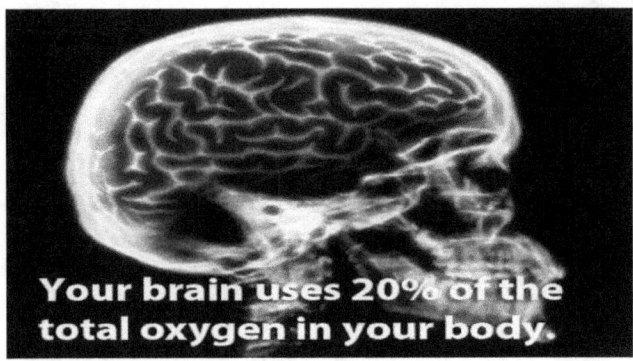

*****Un-Balanced Nervous System**. Lack-of/Low **Oxygen** creates **STRESS**, making our Bodies attempt to **Breathe** Harder/Faster to compensate by attempting to take-in More **Air**, BUT only causing more **Total Body Stress**.

*****Bad HEART/Constricted Blood Vessels**. The **Heart** is constantly beating at an approximate Rate of **80** beats a minute = **4,800** beats per hour = **115,200** beats a day = **42,048,000** beats a year. Making the **Heart** a HUGE consumer of **Oxygen**.

Lack-of/Low **Oxygen** creates a Weak/Slow Heart Beat/Pressure = Poor Total **Body Life-Blood** Circulation = Poor/weak total **Body** Health.

*Less **ENERGY**. Improper Breathing lessens the **Body's** abilities to deliver **Oxygen** to our **CELLS**.

The **Cells** become stressed and have to go into Survival Mode instead of **GROWTH** and **DEVELOPMENT**.

Other Negative Effects Include, but are not limited to :

*Poor Concentration

*Easily Stressed and Anxious

*Shortness of Breath when moving SHORT distances/periods

*Cramping of LEG muscles

*Swollen ANKLES

*General Fatigue

*Re-Occurring CHEST Infection

The **Above** listed Ailments are the **Direct EFFECTS** created from the **Direct CAUSE** of **NOT Breathing** as created – in accordance with the **Laws** of **Respiration**.

'**CAUSE and EFFECT**' is a constant and consistent **Law** that is Applied regardless of Race, Class or Creed.

The **Breath Of LIFE** in the **Atomic** form of **Oxygen** is the **FUEL** source for our **Bodies**.

Oxygen is utilized for **Cellular Restoration**. **Cellular Restoration** is the Process **Cells** use to retrieve the **Energy** stored IN **Carbohydrates** (as well as other foods) and convert those **Carbohydrates** INTO **Energy**. **Lack** of **Oxygen** hampers/prevents the break-down of **Carbohydrates** = production of **Body FAT** !

OxyGen ... The Breath Of Life In Atomic Form!

Obesity is a **Direct EFFECT**, produced from the **Direct CAUSE** of **NOT Breathing** as Created – **Nose** & **Diaphragm** - in accordance with the **Laws** of **Respiration**.

The Natural **CAUSE** of **Breathing** as **Created** produces the Natural **EFFECT** of a **High Metabolism** – **NO FAT** !!

Oxygen is a **Highly Flammable Substance** that Increases **Chemical Reactions**. In our **Bodies**,

Oxygen Thins the **Blood**, which helps to Lower and Regulate **Blood Pressure** and Maximize **Speed** and **Flow**. This Naturally Increases our Rate of **Metabolism** and **Burns** more **Fats/Calories**.

Our **Bodies** uses **HEAT** to create/provide its necessary **Energy** to Move, Function and Live…

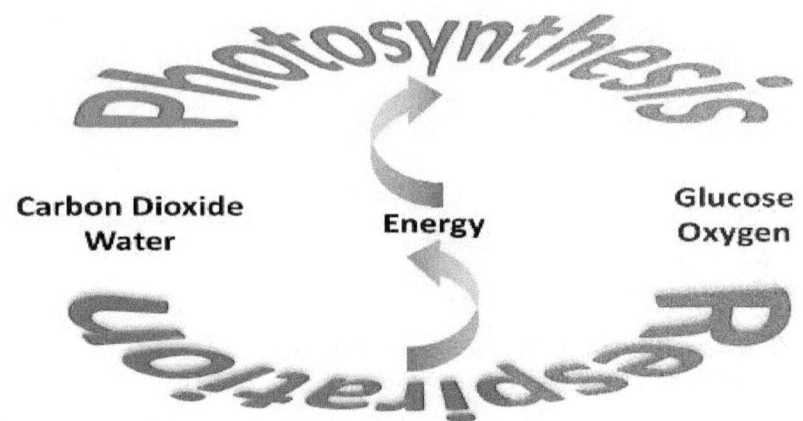

Everything in **Life** is Created of **ATOMS**, so everything involves the **Science** of **Atomic Reactions**. Understanding the **Laws** that Govern **Atomic Reactions** = Understanding the **Laws** that Govern **Self**.

OxyGen ... The Breath Of Life In Atomic Form!

Individual **Atomic Particles** are **Bonded** together to Form **Us**. Understanding **Atomic Bonds** and the **Laws** that Govern them = Understanding the very Fabric of Our Own **Atomic Self**....as we NEED those **Bonds** to BE **Us**.

It is in the **Breaking** of **Atomic Bonds** in the **Foods** and Drinks consumed, that supply the necessary **Energy** to produce and perform the **Function** of LIFE = **Cellular Respiration**.

Cellular Respiration is the **Process** that our **Cells** under-go in utilizing the **Breath** of **LIFE** as starting **Energy** to adequately **Process** and **Create** (Breaking Food Bonds release and creating new ones to gather Waste) **ENERGY** from the **Foods** we eat.

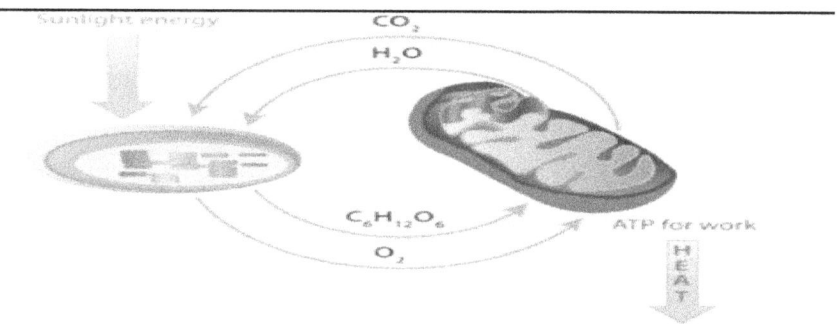

Photosynthesis
- It takes place in a chloroplast.
- Carbon dioxide and water react using light energy, to produce glucose and oxygen.
- Light energy from the sun changes to chemical energy in glucose.

Cellular respiration
- It takes place in a mitochondrion.
- Glucose and oxygen react to produce carbon dioxide, water, and energy (ATP).
- Chemical energy in glucose changes to chemical energy in ATP.

Breathing as **Created** is the **ONLY** way to supply the necessary amount of **Oxygen** needed for this **Process** that is the **Foundation** of our **LIFE**.

Even though **Oxygen** is invisible to the Naked-eye, its Composition is no different – **Atoms** Bonded Together.

OxyGen ... The Breath Of Life In Atomic Form!

Atomic Bonds can be broken either **Chemically** or **Physically**. When **Atomic Bonds** are Broken = Release of **Atomic Energy/Power**. This is the simplistic Function of a **Atomic/Nuclear Reactor**. This is the process that our **LUNGS** take **Oxygen** through when we Breathe.

We **Inhale** the Atomic Molecule **Oxygen (O2)** and **Exhale** the Atomic Molecule **CARBON DIOXIDE (CO2)**. So, our **Lungs** Separate the **Atomic** Composition of **Oxygen** – Separating the **2 Oxygen Atoms**, therein **RELEASING** the **Atomic ENERGY**.

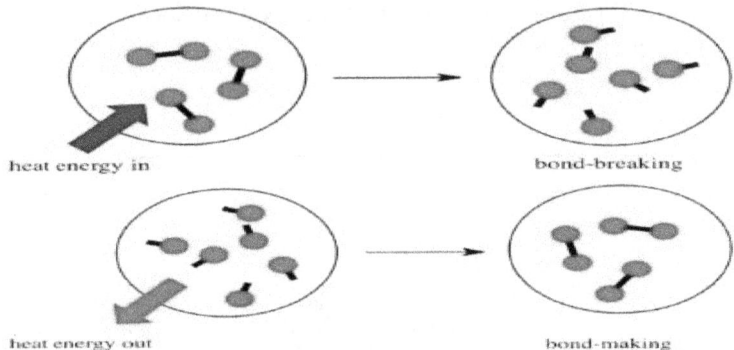

heat energy in   bond-breaking

heat energy out   bond-making

Our **Cells** use the **Energy** released from the broken Bonds of Oxygen to Metabolize **Glucose** = Creating **Energy** to Re-Generate.

The newly separated **Oxygen Atoms** - instantaneously **Bond** with the **Atomic Energy** Waste – manifested in the form of **Carbon**, creating **CO2**.

Energy of Covalent Bonds

Bond	Amount of energy
C – C	82.7 Kcal / mol
C – O	83.9
O = O	96.1
C – H	98.7
O – H	110.7
C = C	147.0
C = O	170
C ≡ C	194

C stands for carbon; O oxygen; H hydrogen.
- indicates a single bond; = a double bond; ≡ a triple bond

OxyGen ... The Breath Of Life In Atomic Form!

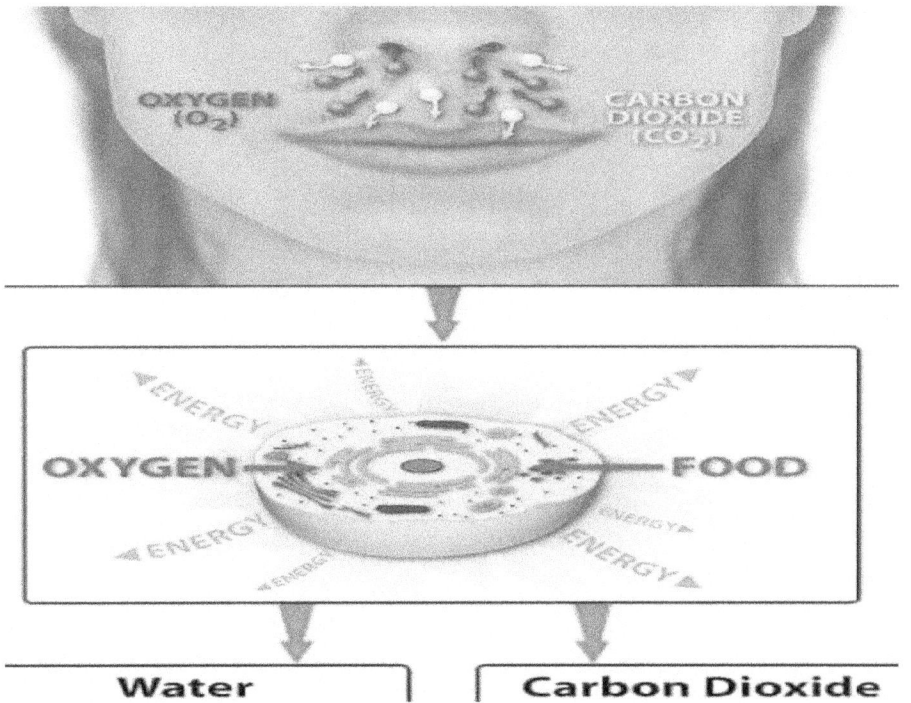

We Use this ENERGY to Move, Talk and LIVE !

OxyGen ... The Breath Of Life In Atomic Form!

Chapter 4 ..... Respiratory System

*****

Every **LIFE** Form is Created with a specific and perfected **Respiratory System** to allow them to Extract the **Breath Of LIFE** (in the form of **Oxygen**) from the **Air** to LIVE.

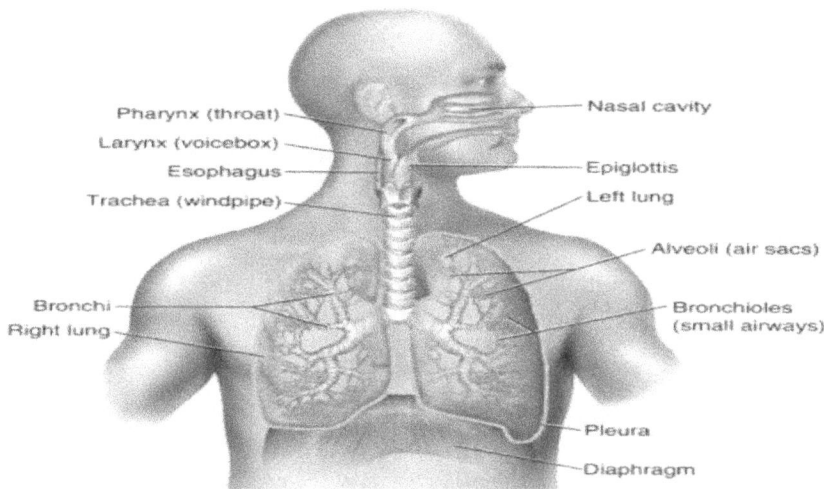

<u>THE MOUTH IS NOT INCLUDED IN THE RESPIRATORY SYSTEM.</u>

We have a Self-Regulating, Natural Breathing Rhythm that's designed to Extract the Maximum amount of **Breath Of LIFE** (**21%** of every **Inhale**) to provide the Proper level of the **Oxygen** to Accomplish any Task, while having the Abilities to Meet and Over-come any and all obstacles in our Path.

Our **Respiratory System** begins in the **Medulla** and **Pons** section of the **Brain**-Stem. Every **Organ** or System of our **Bodies** is controlled by a specific section of our **Brains**.

OxyGen ... The Breath Of Life In Atomic Form!

Our **Brains -** naturally and rhythmically - coordinate our Breathing to/with any activity – ensuring that we have optimal Energy for Success !

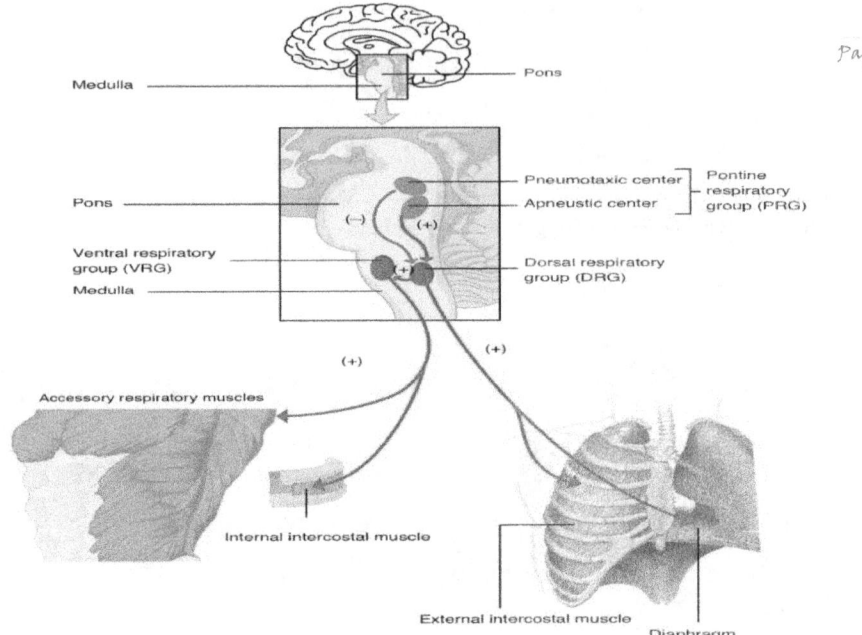

The Center of our **Respiratory** System is in the **Ventral (VRG), Dorsal (DRG)** and **Pontine (PRG) Respiratory** Groups.

The **VRG** controls our **Internal Intercostal Muscles** and **Accessory Respiratory Muscles** that control our **Chest** and **Abdominal** muscles to **Expand** and **Contract** = **Breathing**.

The **PRG** group controls the **DRG** group. The **DRG** group controls our **Diaphragm** and **External Intercostal Muscles**.

Our **Respiratory** System is designed to KEEP us Alive !!!!

OxyGen ... The Breath Of Life In Atomic Form!

Whenever there is a build-up of **Carbon Dioxide** (CO_2), which comes from using the **Mouth** and **Holding Breath**, the DRG and VRG groups automatically **MAKE** us **Breathe** to preserve our LIFE

The **Respiratory** System is apart of the **In—Voluntary** system, but can be manipulated by us. Unfortunately, when we interfere it's usually in a detrimental fashion. When we interfere, we use the **MOUTH** !!!

THE MOUTH IS NOT INCLUDED IN THE RESPIRATORY SYSTEM !!

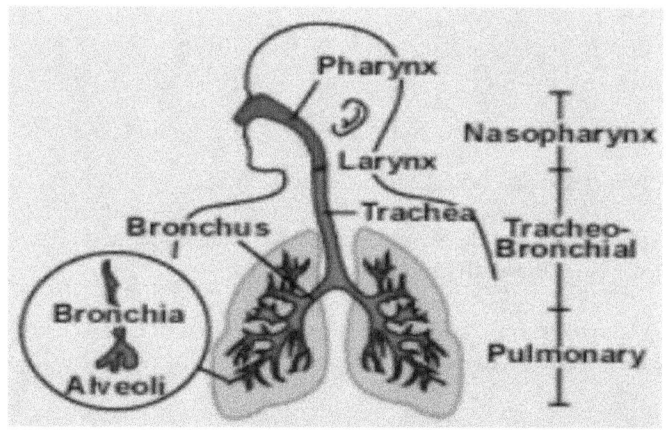

When we use our **Mouth** to Breathe – we are causing instant damage to our **Respiratory Tract** and **System**. The longer we use the **Mouth** = Causing Irreparable Damage.

The **PHARYNX** is the Beginning and End of the **Respiratory** System. The **Pharynx** is connected too the **Nasal Cavity**.

As the **Mouth** is the 1st beginning of our **Digestive** System, using it to Breathe destroys **Nerves**, **Saliva Glands** and **Taste Buds**.

The **Respiratory** System is broken-down into 2 parts – **Upper** & **Lower Respiratory Tracts**.

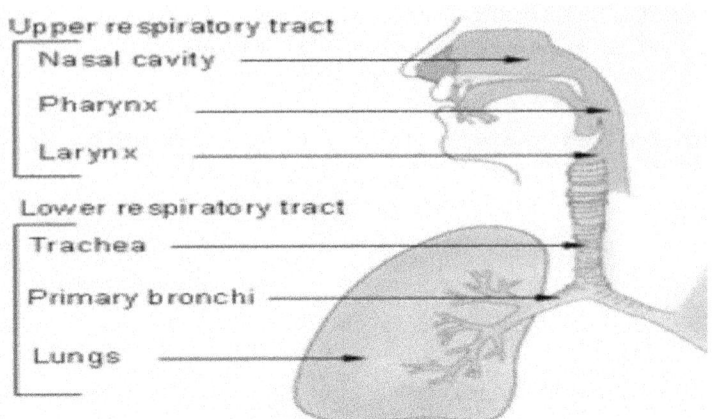

THE MOUTH IS NOT INCLUDED IN THE RESPIRATORY SYSTEM !!

Our **Respiratory System** Begins and Ends with the **Nose**. The **Upper Respiratory System** represents the Entrance and Exit for the **Breath Of LIFE**.

The **Biblical** Scripture states the **GOD** used our **Nostrils/Nose** to place the **Breath Of LIFE** into us. That process established the **Laws** for our **Respiratory System**.

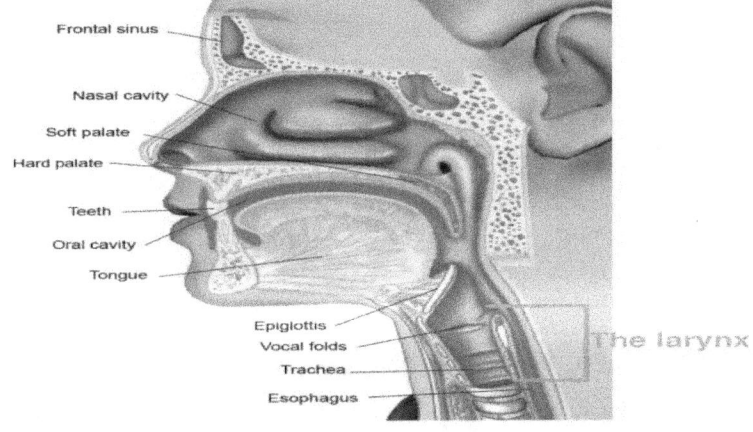

OxyGen ... The Breath Of Life In Atomic Form!

In the Womb, our **Lower Respiratory System** starts to be Created at the start of the 4th week.

Starting with the **Pharynx (Throat)**, the **Laryngotracheal Tube** and **Splanchnic Mesoderm** begin to form the **Trachea Tube (Respiratory** passage).

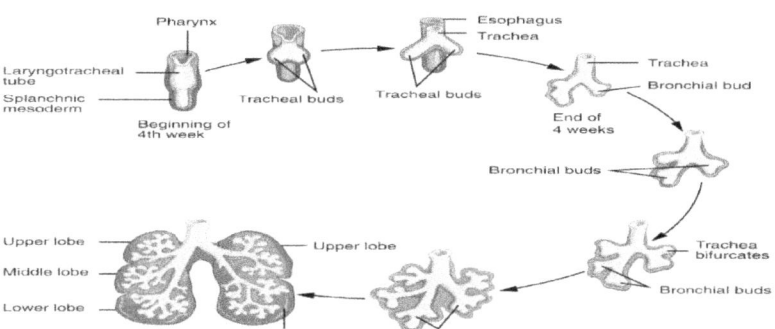

At the end of the 4th week, the **Pharynx** is separated and the **Esophagus (Digestive** System) and the **Trachea (Respiratory** System) are formed.

At the end of 8 weeks, we have the formation of all the **Lobes** that comprise our **Lungs**.

The **Esophagus** and **Trachea** are separated by the **Epiglottis**. The **Epiglottis** protects the **Trachea** when we **Swallow**.

The **Trachea** (also called **Windpipe**) is the most important part of our **Respiratory System**. It's a strong, wide Tube for transporting **Air** to the **Bronchi**. The **Esophagus** is the link between the **Mouth** an **Stomach**. Its smaller and more flexible.

Blood is supplied to each differently. The **Trachea** is supplied by the **Inferior Thyroid Arteries**. The **Esophagus** – by the **Arteries** in the **Neck**, **Thorax** and **Abdomen**

The **Trachea** is comprised of 2 parts – **Thoracic** parts and **Cervical** parts.

The **Esophagus** is comprised of 3 parts – **Thoracic** parts, **Cervical** parts and **Abdominal** parts.

OxyGen ... The Breath Of Life In Atomic Form!

The **Laryngotracheal Tube** forms the base for the **Trachea**. The **Splanchnic Mesoderm** forms the base for the **Bronchial Tubes** – which are the foundation of our **Respiratory** System.

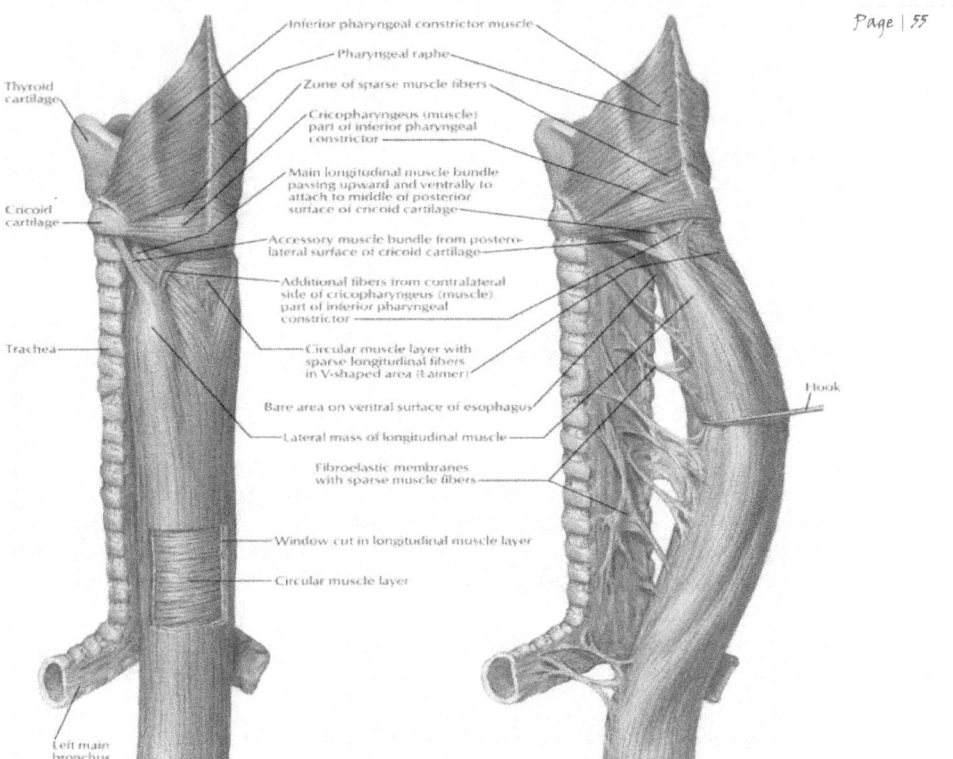

Musculature of Esophagus

The **Trachea** and **Bronchial Tubes** are start of the **Lower Respiratory Tract**. They are the passages that move the **Breath Of LIFE** into the **LUNGS**.

OxyGen ... The Breath Of Life In Atomic Form!

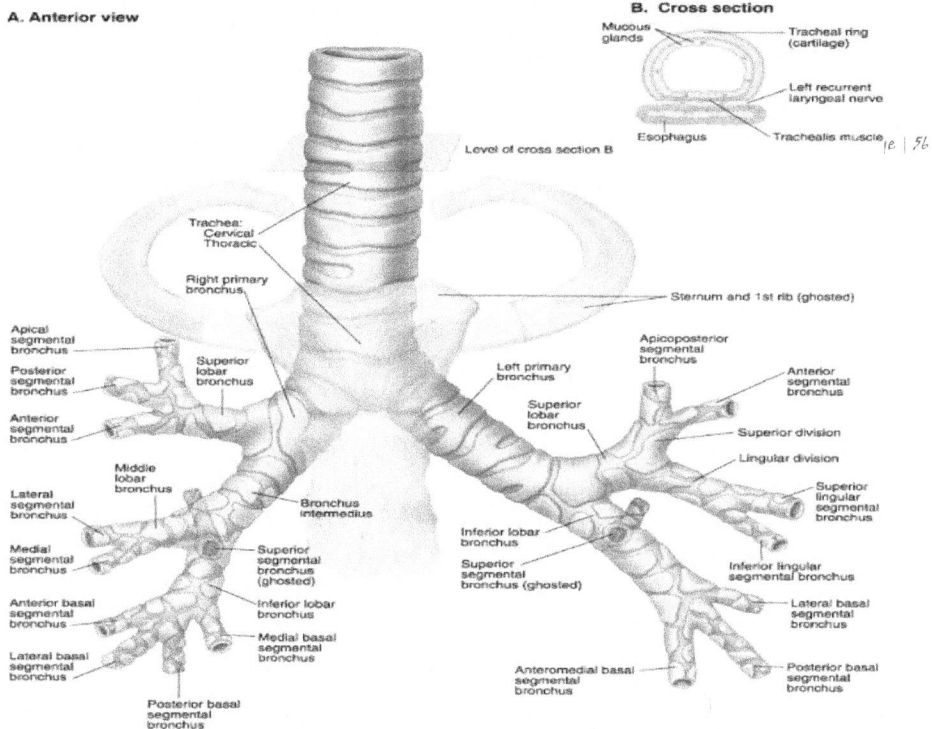

The **Bronchial Tubes** are broken-down into 3 main sections – Left & Right **Main** (primary) **Bronchus**, Left & Right **Lobar** (secondary) **Bronchus** and Left & Right **Segmental** (tertiary) **Bronchus**.

The **Segmental Bronchus** carries the breath of **Air** to the **Bronchiole**. From the **Bronchiole**, the breath goes to the **Terminal Bronchiole**, where the **Alveoli** prepares the **Breath Of LIFE** in the form of **Oxygen** to be extracted and utilized.

OxyGen ... The Breath Of Life In Atomic Form!

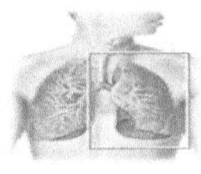
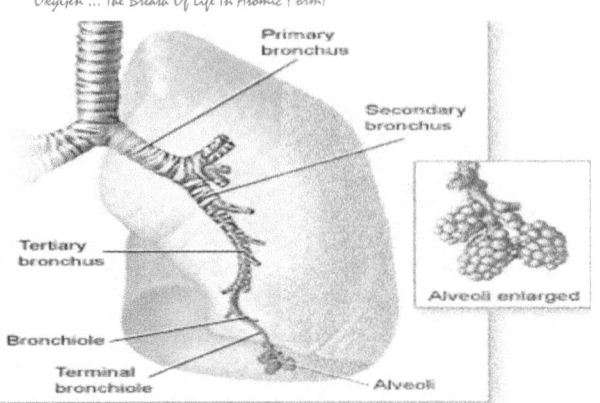

These **3** sections of the **Bronchial Tube** are also responsible for providing **Oxygen** to the **3** main sections of the **Lungs** – Left & Right **Lungs Superior Lobes**, Right **Lung Middle Lobe** and Left & Right **Lungs Inferior Lobes**.

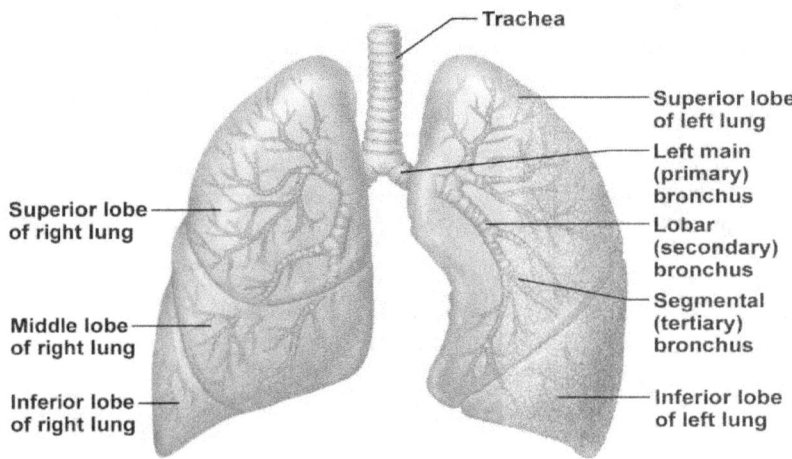

We are Created with a Perfectly functional and operating Respiratory System that is designed to keep us HERE in this Physical level of existence for a VERY LONG TIME!!!!

All we have to dp is simply Breathe As CREATED!

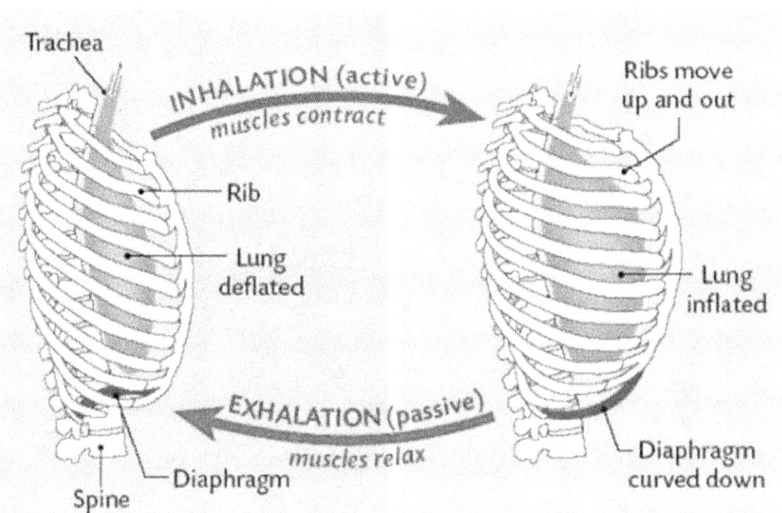

OxyGen ... The Breath Of Life In Atomic Form!

Chapter 5 ..... How Our Lungs Work

*****

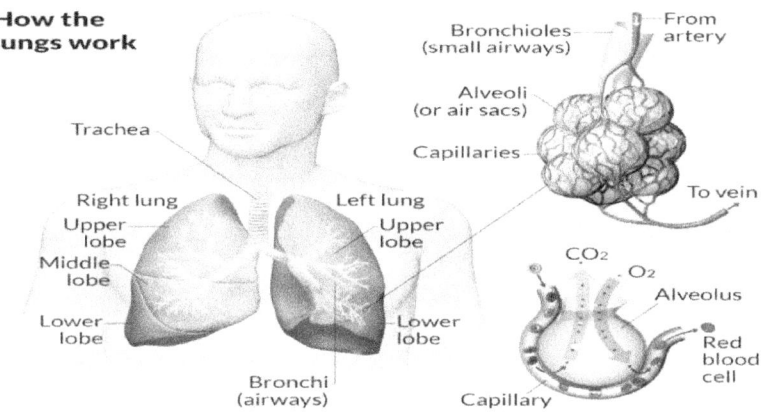

Every **Inhaled** Breath sends the **Air** to the **Alveolus.**

The **Alveoli** are the **Respiratory**

Membranes where the **Breath Of LIFE** is prepared to be Extracted.

The **Alveoli** are lined with **Capillaries**.

OxyGen ... The Breath Of Life In Atomic Form!

Respiratory Membrane

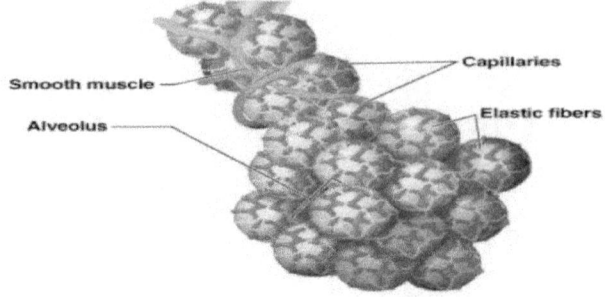

The **Capillaries** are where the **Breath Of LIFE** is Diffused and **Carbon Dioxide** Removed.

Oxygen and **Carbon Dioxide** are exchanged thru the **Capillaries**.

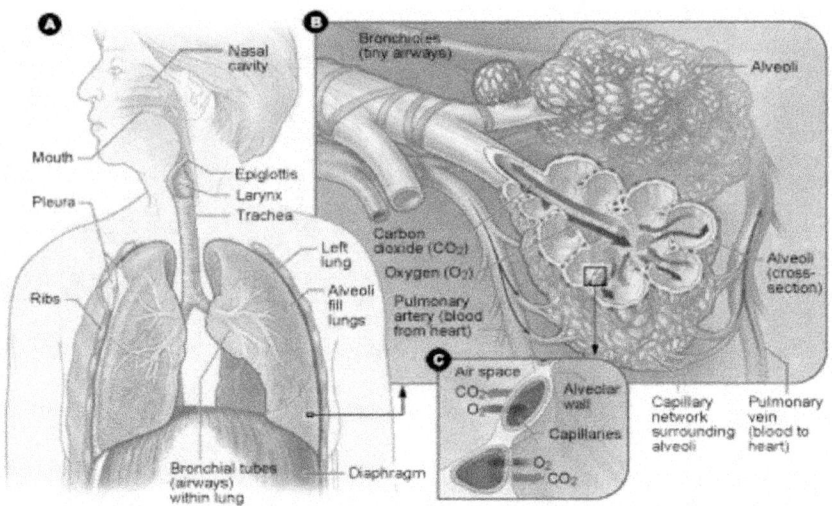

Because the **Capillaries** are deep within the **Lungs**, proper **Breathing** (**Diaphragm**) is vital to achieving a Full, Deep **Breath Of LIFE** !

So, it's IMPERATIVE that we ALWAYS **Breath** as **Created**, which Naturally maintains our **Oxygen** Composition = BE WHO WE ARE CREATED TO BE !

Chest Breathing only provides Shallow, Half Breaths = Less **Oxygen** = Other-than Our **Atomic** Self.

Not **Breathing** as Created is the **Cause** that produces the Negative **Effect** of NOT having the Proper **Oxygen** Ratio = sicknesses, dis-eases and pre-mature death.

OxyGen ... The Breath Of Life In Atomic Form!

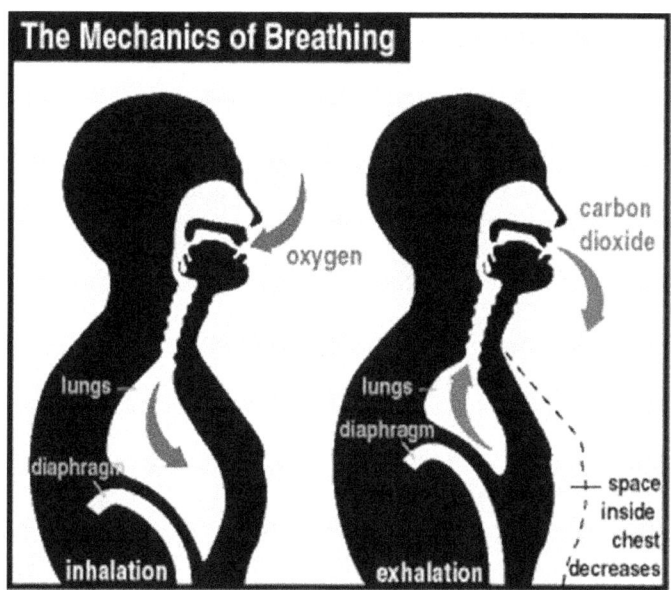

OxyGen ... The Breath Of Life In Atomic Form!

Chapter 6 ...... Pulmonary Ventilation

******

Pulmonary Ventilation is the act of **Breathing**. **Breathing** is the commonly used term for **VENTILATION** and **RESPIRATION** or the **RESPIRATION** Cycle

Ventilation is the process of **INSPIRATION** (Oxygen IN) and **EXPIRATION** (Oxygen OUT) of the **Lungs**.

We **Breathe** for the purpose of getting **Oxygen** IN our **Body** and **Carbon Dioxide** OUT. Our **Cells** need **Oxygen** to make the **Energy**-containing **Molecule ATP**. **Carbon Dioxide** is the byproduct of **ATP Synthesis**.

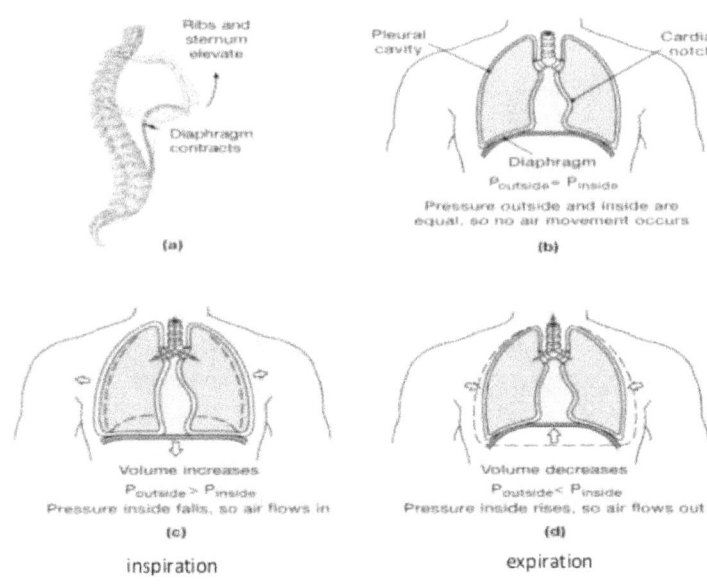

OxyGen ... The Breath Of Life In Atomic Form!

The ability to **Breathe** is dependent on the **Air Pressure** between the **Atmosphere** and our **Lungs**.

The major mechanisms that drive **Pulmonary Ventilation** are – **Atmospheric** Pressure (**Patm**), **Alveolar** Pressure (**Palv**) – Pressure within the **Alveoli** and **Intrapleural** Pressure (**Pip**) – Pressure within the **Pleural Cavity**.

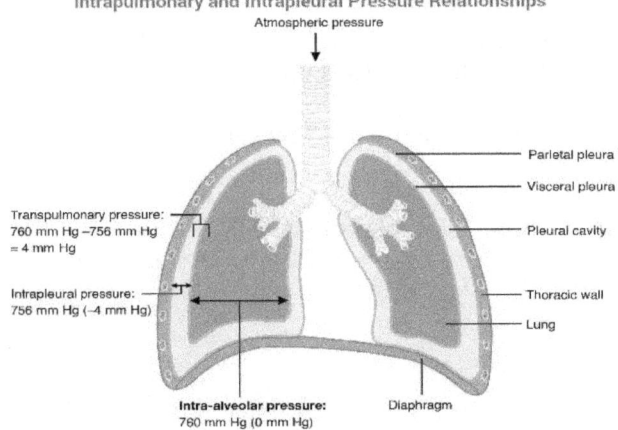

Figure 2. Alveolar pressure changes during the different phases of the cycle. It equalizes at 760 mm Hg but does not remain at 760 mm Hg.

Inspiration occurs when **Lung Pressure** is DECREASED BELOW Atmospheric Pressure, which causes **Air IN**.

Expiration occur when **Lung Pressure** is INCREASED ABOVE Atmospheric Pressure – which **Pushes Air OUT**.

Atmospheric Pressure is the amount of **Force** exerted on our Bodies by the Air surrounding us. For our **Respiration**, the **Negative** (Lower-than) and the **Positive** (Higher-than) **Pressures** are the main components.

Intra-Alveolar Pressure is the pressure of the **Air** in the **Alveoli**, which changes during the different phases of **Breathing**. Because the **Alveoli** are connected to the **Atmosphere**, the **Intrapulmonary Pressure** in them equalizes with the **Atmospheric Pressure**.

OxyGen ... The Breath Of Life In Atomic Form!

Intrapleural Pressure is the pressure of the **Air** within the **Pleural Cavity,** between the **Visceral** and **Parietal Pleural**. The **Intrapleural Pressure** is always **Negative** (Lower) to **Atmospheric Pressure.**

Boyles Law is the reference of the processes of **Gases** under **Scientific Law**. **Boyles Law** states that, the **Pressure** of a **Container** of **Gas DECREASES** as the **Volume** of the **Container INCREASES**.

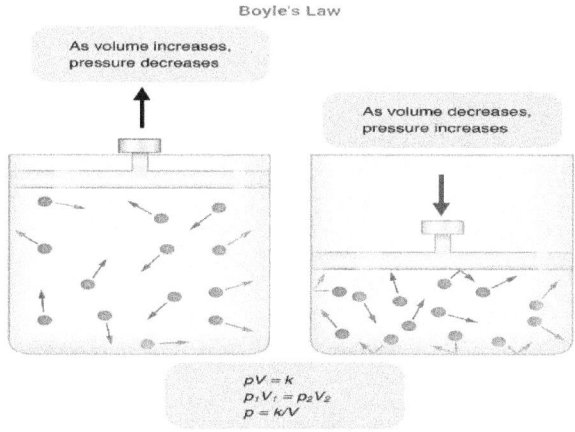

Figure 1. In a gas, pressure increases as volume decreases.

Our **Lungs** are similar to a **Container** and fall under the same **Laws**. When **Lung Pressure** or **Intra-Pulmonary Pressure** becomes **LESS** than **Atmospheric Pressure** – this creates a **Pressure Gradient**.

With the **Nose OPEN**, **Air** moves **INTO** the **Lungs** until the **Pressure** Equilibrates.

There are **3 Processes Essential** for the transfer of **Oxygen** from the outside **Air** to the **Blood** flowing thru the **Lungs** – **VENTILATION, DIFFUSION** and **PERFUSION**.

Ventilation is the process by which **Air** moves **In** and **Out** of our **Lungs**.

OxyGen ... The Breath Of Life In Atomic Form!

Diffusion is the spontaneous movement of **Gases** without the use of **Energy** or **Effort** by the Body. **Diffusion** happens between the **Gas** in the **Alveoli** and the **Blood** in the **Capillaries** in the **Lungs**.

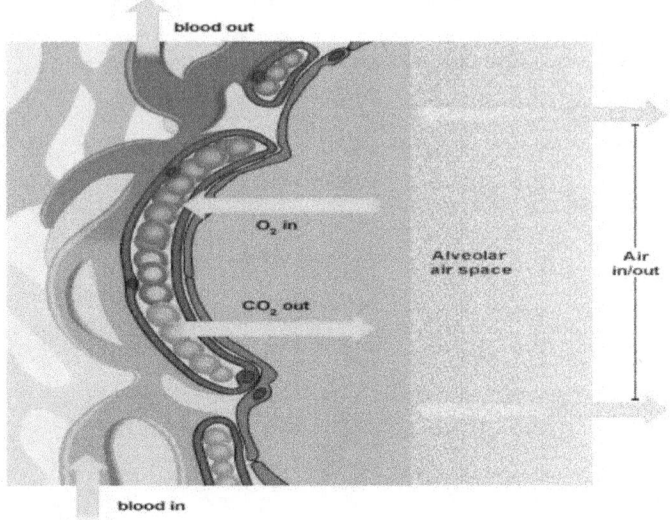

Perfusion is the process by which the **Cardiovascular System** pumps **Blood** throughout the **Lungs**.

Breathing Effects us in different ways. The **BRAIN** requires **20%** of inhaled **Oxygen**, the most of any **Organ**/System, so the **BRAIN** is **Oxygen** Dependent.

The **Inhaled Breath** goes into our **Lungs**. From the **Lungs**, the **Arteries** absorb the **Oxygen** (O2) and carries **FRESH Oxygenated Blood** to the **Cells** of our **Body**. Each **Cell** uses the **Oxygen** to 'BURN' as **Fuel** to generate **Energy**. As the **Oxygen** is burned/used up **Carbon Dioxide** (CO2) is produced.

The **Carbon Dioxide** and any remaining **Oxygen** are collected by our **Blood** and transported thru the **Veins** BACK into the **Lungs** to be **Exhaled OUT**.

There is approximately **14.7 Pounds** of **Atmospheric Pressure Per Square** Inch of Body surface. **Breathing Equalizes** the OutSide **1 Tonnage** of **Atmospheric Pressure** with the **Pressure** InSide of us = allowing us to **NOT** be **Crushed**.

Breathing is 1ˢᵗ part of the **Physiological Respiration REQUIRED** to sustain **Life**. The **Oxygen** extracted from each **Breath** produces the **Energy** required for the Functions of Life.

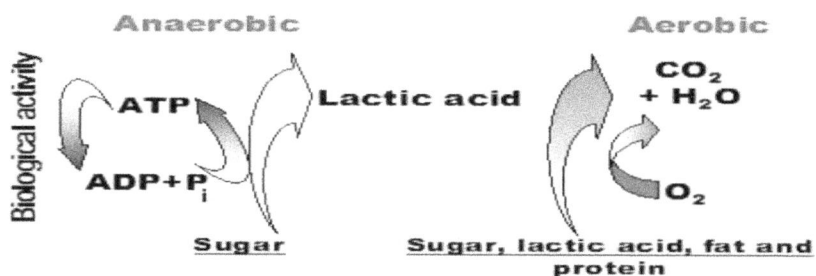

Humans are **AEROBIC** Organisms that **REQUIRE** Oxygen to release **Energy** via **Cellular Respiration**.

AEROBIC means **WITH** Oxygen.

*Word equation for **Aerobic Respiration** : Glucose + Oxygen – Carbon Dioxide + Water + Energy.

RESPIRATION

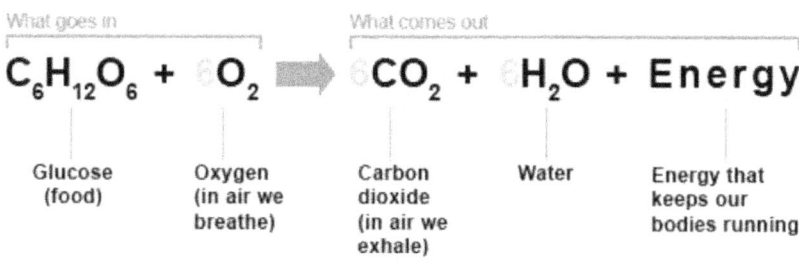

OxyGen ... The Breath Of Life In Atomic Form!

ANAEROBIC is the Opposite of **Aerobic**, meaning **WITHOUT** Oxygen.

*Word Equation for **Anaerobic Respiration** : Glucose - Lactic Acid + Energy.

> Energy from glucose is obtained from the oxidation reaction
> $$C_6H_{12}O_6 + 6O_2 \longrightarrow 6CO_2 + 6H_2O$$

Humans are **Herbivores**. **GLUCOSE** is an Energy-Rich **Molecule** that is Our **Cellular** Food.

Glucose is the Primary **Molecule** produced by **Fruits** & **Veggies** that our Bodies convert into **Energy**. **Oxygen** is the catalyst that produces the **METABOLIC Reaction** to break down **Glucose**. This Process creates the **ENERGY/POWER** that we Use to **LIVE/Move**.

GLUCLOSE is the **FOOD** of **LIFE** !

Glucose is a **Molecule** that's also considered - the **Natural Sugar** of **Life**.

Glucose is the Natural Occurring process of **Energy** provided through Food. Our Bodies uses **Glucose** to Feed and Replenish its **Energy**. When we **Inhale Oxygen**, our **Lungs** separate the **Atoms**....that **Power** that is released, provides **Energy** in the Form of **HEAT**.

This **HEAT** then works to **Decompose** the **GLUCOSE**, turning the potential Harmful **Sugars** of **Glucose** into **WATER** and **CARBON DIOXIDE**. The **Water** is Absorbed by our **Bodies** and travel with **Carbon Dioxide** when it's **Exhaled OUT**.

Biomedical Importance Of Glucose

- Glucose is a major carbohydrate
- It is a major fuel of tissues
- It is converted into other carbohydrates
  - ✓ Glycogen for storage.
  - ✓ Ribose in nucleic acids.
  - ✓ Galactose in lactose of milk.
  - ✓ They form glycoproteins & proteoglycans
  - ✓ They are present in some lipoproteins (LDL) .
  - ✓ Present in plasma membrane;glycocalyx.
  - ✓ Glycophorin is a major intergral membrane glycoprotein of human erythrocytes.

The **Oxygen Molecule** is the Catalyst to Successfully transforming Our **Foods** INTO **Energy**, while simultaneously eliminating the Waste.

OxyGen ... The Breath Of Life In Atomic Form!

Breathing is also the act of **Gas Exchange**. Providing Fresh, Pure **Oxygen** while simultaneously Removing **Carbon Dioxide** and Excess **Water**/Vapor.

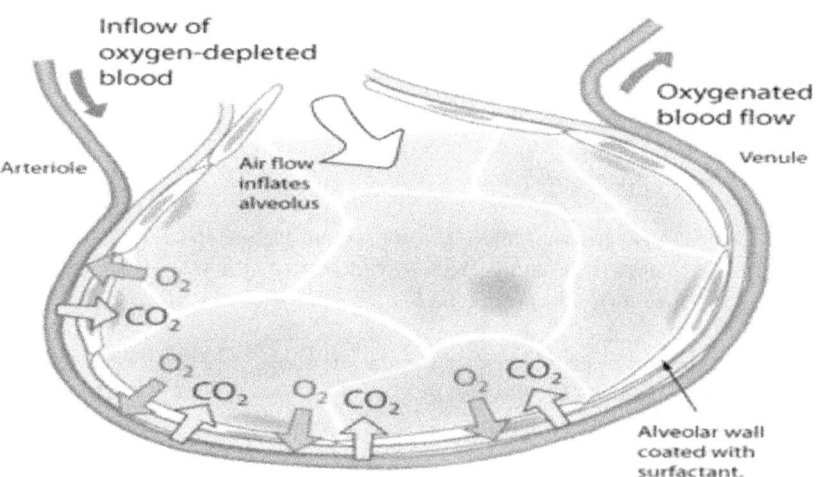

As **Oxygen** enters the **Lungs**, it is diffused in the **Alveoli**. The **Alveoli** allow the **Oxygen** to be infused with the **Hemoglobin** in **Red Blood Cells** and carried thru the **Bloodstream** around the **Body**.

When it reaches a **Cell** requiring **Oxygen** – it Diffuses into the **Cell**.

The **Cells** break the **Covalent Bonds** of **Oxygen** to release it's **Energy** for use.

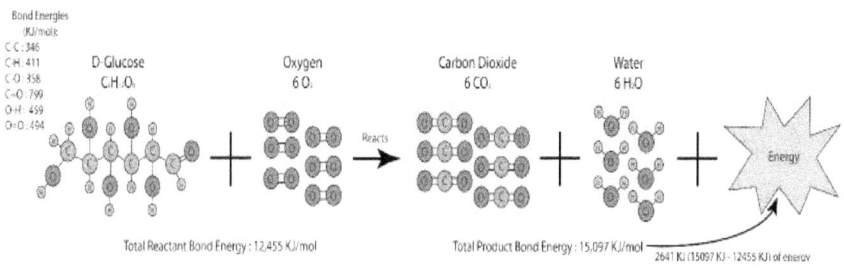

OxyGen ... The Breath Of Life In Atomic Form!

When **Atomic Bonds** are broken – **New** ones are IMMEDIATELY Formed. So, when **Oxygen** is Diffused **INTO** the **Cells** – the **Carbon** (Respiratory waste) is Diffused **OUT** of the **Cells** and **Bonds** to the newly broken **Oxygen Molecule** to form **Carbon Dioxide**. This is infused in the **Hemoglobin** and carried in the **Bloodstream**, back to the **Lungs** to be **Exhaled OUT**.

The **Air** we Breathe **IN** has **21%** **Oxygen** (O2) and **0.04%** **Carbon Dioxide** (CO2).

The **Air** we Breathe **OUT** has **17%** **Oxygen** (O2) and **4%** **Carbon Dioxide** (CO2).

We were Created with a Natural Self-Regulating **Respiratory** System.

Breathing is Controlled by specialized centers in the **Brain-Stem**. When **Carbon Dioxide** levels increase in the **Blood**, it Reacts with the **Water** in the **Blood** creating **CARBONIC Acid**. This **LOWERS** the **PH** (**Potential/Power** of **Hydrogen**) of our **Bodies**.

This drop in **PH** Levels triggers **Chemoreceptors** in the **Carotid** and **Aortic** Bodies. Also triggering the **Respiratory** center in the **Medulla Oblongata**.

These steps activate our **In-Voluntary** muscles that automatically adjusts (faster/slower) our **Breathing Rhythm**, according to our activities, to Deliver the Proper amount of **Oxygen/Energy**, allowing us to Accomplish any and all Endeavors.

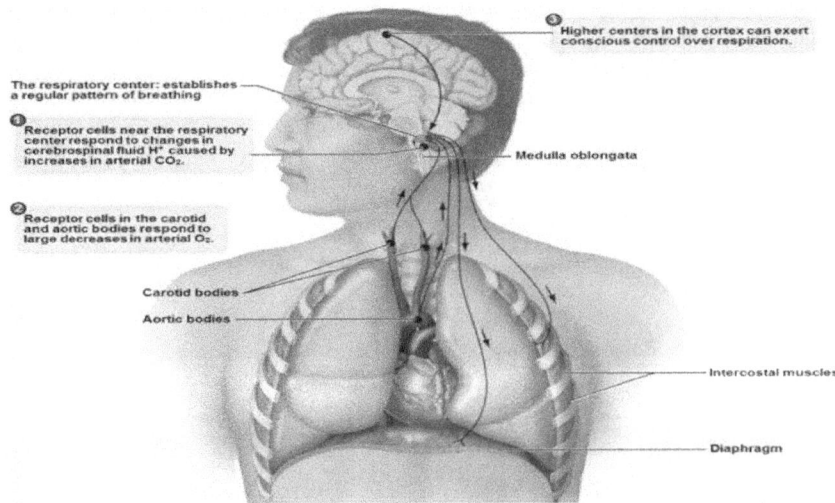

It is a Build-Up of **CARBON DIOXIDE** that makes the **Blood** become **Acidic.**

This in turn causes the sensation of **NEEDING** a **Breath**. The results are an Increase in **Heart** Rate and **Breathing** = **INCREASE** of **STRESS** throughout the entire Body.

HEALTH

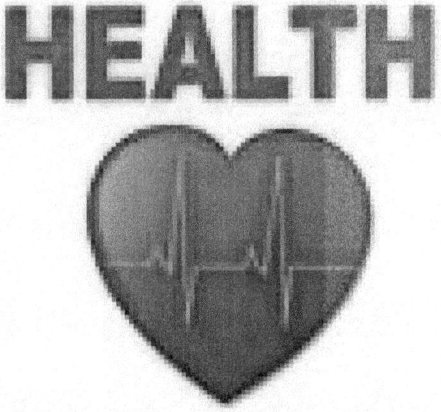

OxyGen ... The Breath Of Life In Atomic Form!

Chapter 7 ...... Hemoglobin

*****

Hemoglobin is an **Iron**-containing **Protein** in **Red Blood Cells** that are responsible for transport of **Oxygen – The Breath Of Life** to the **Tissues/Cells** and removing **Carbon Dioxide** from them.

In the **Lungs** during **Inhaling**, **Hemoglobin** reacts to **Oxygen** and forms **OXYHEMOGLOBIN**. From there, it travels thru the **Bloodstream** to the **Cells**. Then it breaks-down to form **Hemoglobin** and **Oxygen** – and **Oxygen** is then Passed thru to the **Cells**.

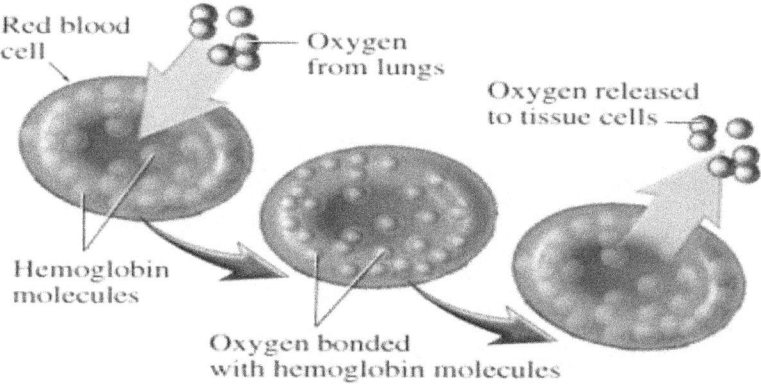

During the **Exhale**, the **Hemoglobin** combines with **Carbon Dioxide** to form **CARBAMINOHEMOGLOBIN**.

Carbaminohemoglobin is an Un-stable compound that Breaks-down to Release the **Carbon Dioxide** OUT of us when we **Exhale**.

OxyGen ... The Breath Of Life In Atomic Form!

Hemoglobin is also commonly referred to as **BLOOD**.

Blood is the **LIFE Water** of our **Physical Bodies**.

§ Blood pressure, resistance, and flow

- **Importance** – deliver oxygen and nutrients and to remove wastes at a rate keeps pace with tissue metabolism
- **Blood flow (F)** – is the amount of blood flowing through an organ, tissue, or blood vessel in a given time
- **Hemodynamics**: Blood Flow (F) = $\Delta P/R$
  – Where ΔP is the pressure difference and R is the resistance

It is thru **Blood, Blood Pressure** and **Blood Flow** that **ALL Nutrition** (Oxygen / Nutrition) **Regulation** of our **Organs** happens. Without the Adequate amount of **Blood, Blood Pressure** and **Blood Flow**, our **Physical Bodies** start to deteriorate (Malnutrition / Oxygen Deficient) to the point of **Pre-Mature Death.**

The **Condition** of **Blood** is **Directly Depend** on the **ADEQUATE AMOUNT OF THE BREATH OF LIFE** (In the Form of **OXYGEN**) !!

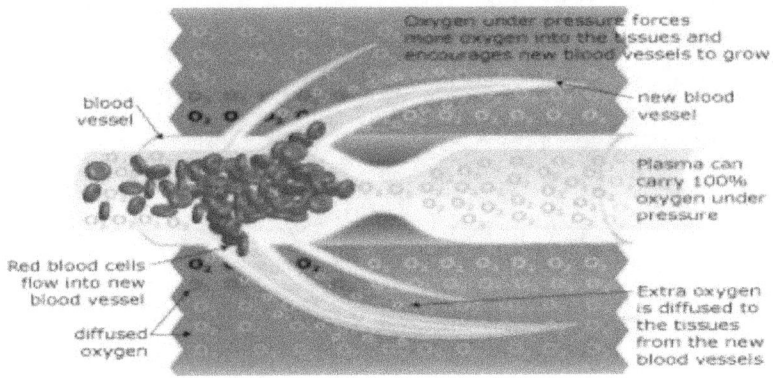

Blood also carries the **Glucose** (**Food** of **LIFE**) needed for **Respiration**. **Glucose** is picked-up by the **Blood Vessels** that surround the **Intestines**. **Glucose** is then carried by the **Blood** to the **Cells** and moves around the **Body**, ensuring that all **Tissues** receive **Oxygen** and **Glucose** for **Energy**.

OxyGen ... The Breath Of Life In Atomic Form!

Blood is mainly **Water**, so it dissolves **Glucose** very well. **Glucose** and **Carbon Dioxide** are dissolved in **PLASMA**. **Plasma** is the **Pale Yellow liquid** part of the **Blood**.

The dissolved **Glucose** diffuses in the **Cells** that need it for **Respiration**.

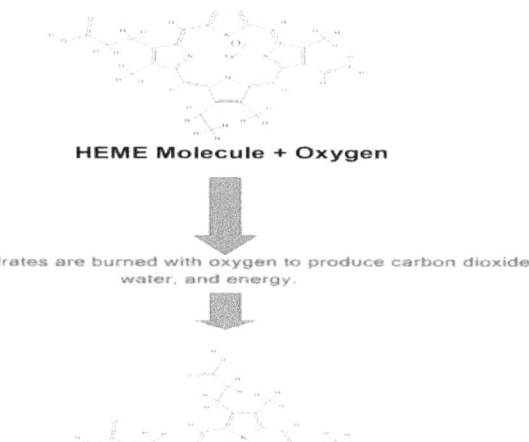

The **Breath Of Life** in the **Atomic** form of **Oxygen** is an Important factor in ALL our **Life** functions. Lack of **Oxygen** or being **Oxygen** deficient impairs the metabolism of **Carbohydrates** and severely decreases **Energy** output and duration.

OxyGen ... The Breath Of Life In Atomic Form!

Chapter 8 ... Diaphragm vs Chest/Thoracic Breathing

*****

The **Diaphragm** is our Natural **Organ** for ensuring a Full, Deep Breath, utilizing the total capacities of the **Lungs** = Adequately supplying Proper **Oxygen** level = Maximum Fuel for

Cellular Respiration = Increased abilities to Build and Maintain **Supreme Health** and **Fitness** !

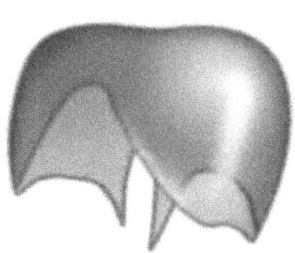

The diaphragm is shaped like a parachute

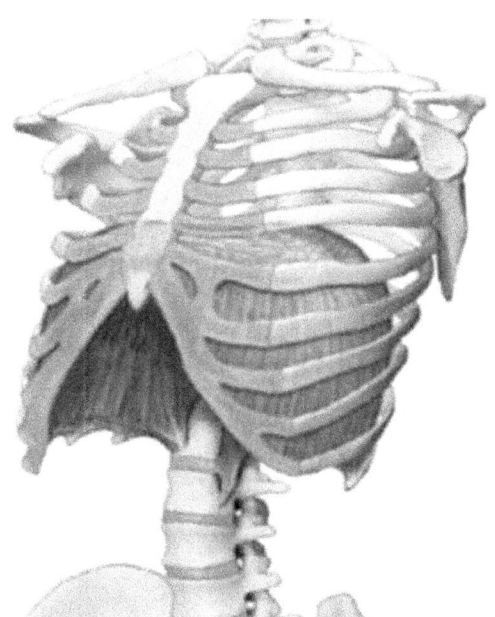

The **Diaphragm** performs the Function of Expanding and Shrinking to Cause the **Lungs** to **Inhale** and **Exhale** (pull-in and push-out Air).

Our Internal Organs operate as independent Systems so we can Function as a Single Unit.

The Diaphragm plays in important function in the overall operations of our internal Systems.

The Nose is the 1st part of the Respiratory system, but utilizing the Diaphragm ensures that we get a FULL Inhalation of the

Breath Of LIFE

The diaphragm moves down when we inhale decreasing pressure on the heart and lungs and increasing pressure on abdominal organs.

The diaphragm moves up when we exhale increasing pressure on the heart and lungs and decreasing pressure on abdominal organs.

The **Diaphragm is the Work Muscle and Engine to proper function and Maximum Inhalation of the Breath Of Life in the Atomic form of Oxygen.**

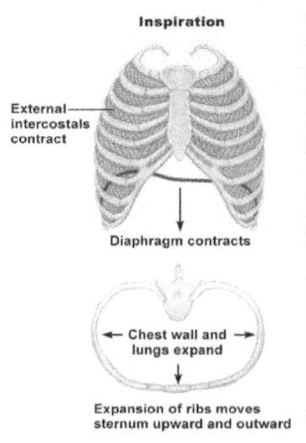

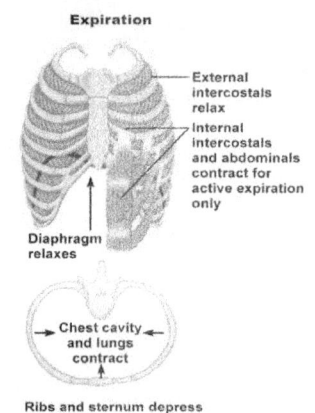

OxyGen ... The Breath Of Life In Atomic Form!

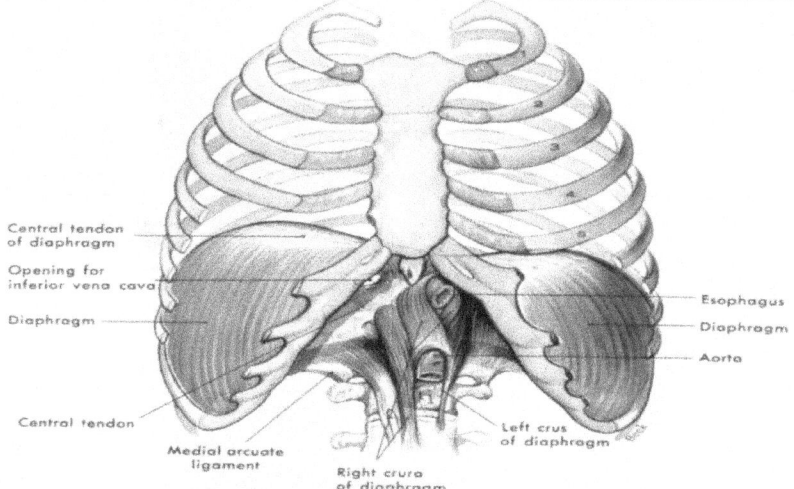

The diaphragm as seen from the front. Note the openings in the vertebral portion for the inferior vena cava, esophagus, and aorta.

Chest Breathing (also called **Thoracic** Breathing) is a Shallow breath, without filling-up and using the full capacities of the **Lungs**. This creates a Low/Deficient **Oxygen** level in Self.

The **CAUSE** of **Chest** breathing produces a dominion type **EFFECT** of cascading Negative Health on all the internal **Organs** and **Systems**.

During times of **Stress**, **Anxiety**, **Anger** and **Fear**, our **Brain** Activates our '*Flight-or-Flight*' Response.

This means our **Bodies** naturally go into **Survival-Defense Mode**. This **Reaction** requires **MORE Oxygen**. To get more **Oxygen**, our **Body** uses the **Chest** to aide the **Diaphragm** in getting more **Air** into the **Lungs**.

This alters the Natural **Ratio/Percentage** of **Oxygen** needed to sustain **Homeostasis**. So, this is a **_TEMPORARY_** State and is designed to be because of the potential harmful side-effects.

Wherein prolonged States of the '**Fight-or-Flight**' Response produces **Free-Radicals** (Un-stable **Atoms**) and creates a Low/Deficient **Oxygen** environment that Dis-eases, Bacteria and Viruses thrive in.

These **Free-Radicals** turn into Dis-eases and **Cancers**, which can only survive in a Low **Oxygen** Environment.

Chest breathing over-utilizes the Breathing Muscles and interferes with our Posture and proper functioning of internal Organs and Systems.

The Head is forced forward, with the Shoulders being forced into a Hunched-up and forward position. This creates an increased sway in the Lower-Back, while simultaneously pushing the Pelvis forward = Mis-Alignment of the entire Body.

Now we have Pain in the Lower-Back and Pelvis areas, while severely decreasing the possibility for Free and Deep Breathing = Deficient/Low Oxygen level in Self = Sicknesses and weakness.

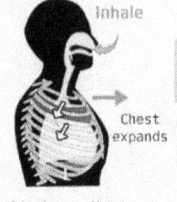

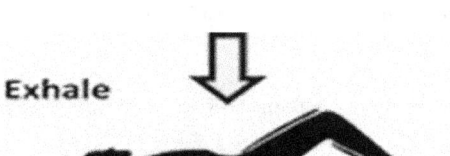

Exhale

Navel draws in toward the spine

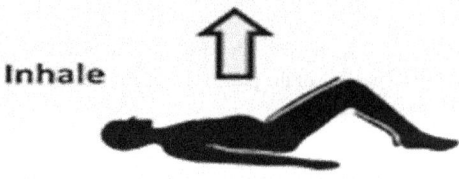

Inhale

Abdomen expands

The Lungs are not like Muscle tissue that move by contractions. They are Sacs that are inflated by the movement of the Diaphragm and deflate from natural pressure.

Proper function of the Lungs is dependent on proper use of the Diaphragm.

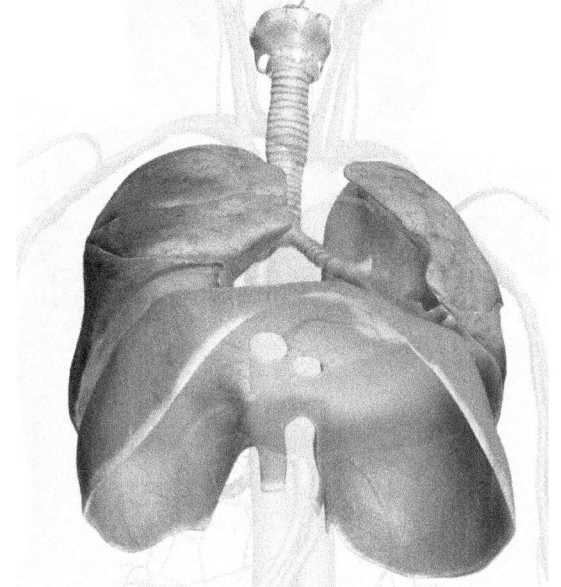

Chapter 9 ...... Nasal vs Mouth Inhalation

*****

The Process of **Inhaling** is also referred to as **Inspiration**.

Our **RESPIRATORY** System **BEGINS** and **ENDS** with our **NOSE** !

Our **MOUTHS** are a part of the **DIGESTIVE** System.

The **Scriptural** description gives **THE CREATOR** using Our **NOSE** to place the **Breath** of **LIFE** into Us. This is the **1st Law** of **Respiration**.

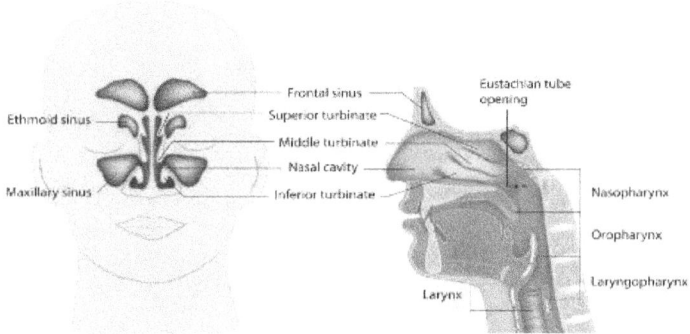

The **Internal Nasal Structure** or **Cavity** houses the system of **Smelling** – **Olfaction** and the top of the **Respiratory** System. The top of the **Nasal** Cavity is directly under the **Brain** and separated by a thin wall of **Bone** and **Mucous Membrane**.

The **Mucous Membrane** contains the **Olfactory Bulb** – which contains millions of **Olfactory Receptor Nerves**. The **Nerves** differentiate between thousands of smells.

OxyGen ... The Breath Of Life In Atomic Form!

The **Nose** is the **Air**-Conditioner and **Filter** for our **Lungs**. The **Cilia** (**Hair**) keeps out dust and microscopic particles.

The **Nasal Cavities** have **Turbinates** (**Shelves**) and **Folds** that warm an add moisture to the **Air** before it reaches the **Lungs**, making **Breathing** much easier.

Inhaling thru the **NOSE** ensures that we receive the Proper **Ratio** of **Oxygen**. Inhaling thru the Nose provides Clean, Warm and Pure Quality of Oxygen that gives the ability to manifest Maximum Energy and Power.

Inhaling thru the **Nose** is the **ONLY** way to achieve and maintain a condition of **Oxygen** Efficiency. Below 96% **Oxygenation** one is scientifically and medically considered **Oxygen** deficient. In a state of being Oxygen deficient, diseases can become present.

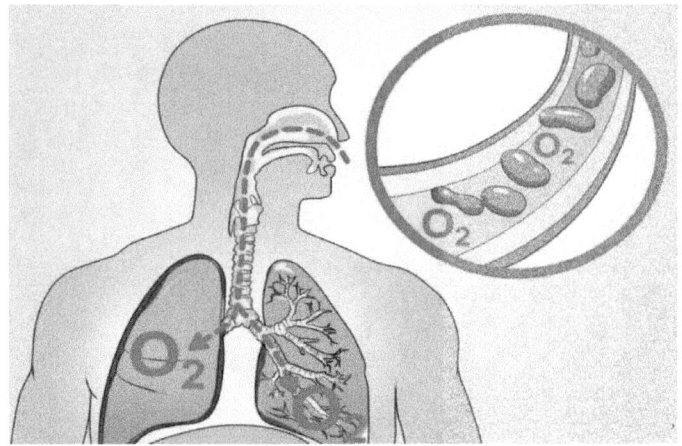

Our **Respiratory** system is perfectly created to transfer the **Atomic Energy** of the **Breath of Life** (**Oxygen**) into the **Power** of **Life**.

Our **Nose's** produce **Nitric Oxide** (**NO**) thru the **Sinus Mucous Membranes** in Small amounts. When **Inhaled**, **Nitric Oxide** (**NO**) significantly Enhances our **Lungs** capacity to absorb **Oxygen** by **10-25%**.

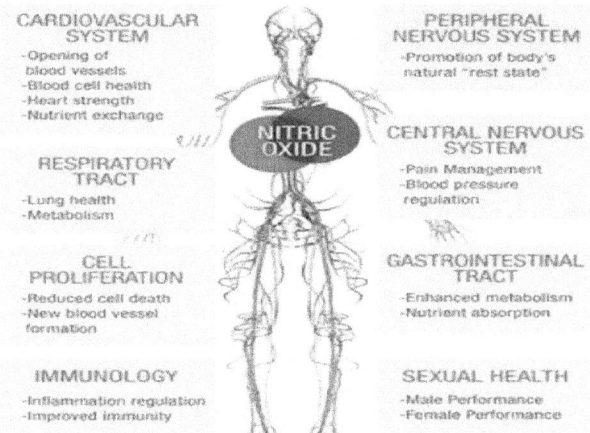

Nitric Oxide (NO) is produced from the stimulation of the 'Bitter Receptors' in Nose's T2R38 Genes. These Receptors react to the Chemicals that Bacteria and Viruses use to Communicate and Grow, becoming Lethal to Bacteria and Viruses = helping to Protect the Lungs and Body.

Nasal Breathing increases Circulation, Blood Oxygen and Carbon Dioxide Levels, while slowing the Breathing Rate and improving overall Lung Volume.

Mouth Breathing leads to Chronic Hyper-Ventilation, Increased levels of Carbon Dioxide, Reduced Blood Circulation, Build-Up of Toxins and Narrowing of Nasal Passages.

Air is Filled with several Pollutants (natural & un-natural), that cause Cellular damage in the form of FREE-RADICALS. Free-Radicals are Atoms that are MISSING an Electron, making them Un-stable.

The NASAL Cavities are Created with necessary Membranes that produce MUCUS (which are able to absorb pollutants), providing CLEAN Oxygen and REDUCING the amount of Harmful Pollutants Inhaled.

Use of the Mouth presents NO Filtering methods. So, Mouth Breathing elevates our Blood Pressure and Heart Rate to Harmful Levels. Mouth Breathing WORSENS Asthma, Allergies, Rhinitis and Sleep Apnea.

OxyGen ... The Breath Of Life In Atomic Form!

WHAT'S IN OUR AIR?

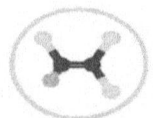 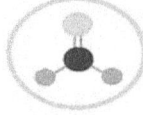  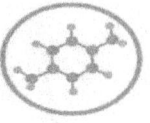 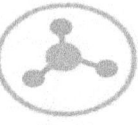

TRICHLOROETHYLENE — Found in printing inks, paints, lacquers, varnishes, adhesives and paint remover/stripper.

FORMALDEHYDE — Found in paper bags, waxed papers, facial tissues, paper towels, table napkins, particle board, plywood panelling, and synthetic fabrics.

BENZENE — Used to make plastics, resins, synthetic fibres, rubber lubricants, dyes, detergents, drugs and pesticides. Can also be found in tobacco smoke, vehicle exhausts, glue, paint and furniture wax.

XYLENE — Found in printing, rubber, leather and paint industries, tobacco smoke and vehicle exhausts.

AMMONIA — Found in window cleaners, floor waxes, smelling salts and fertilizers.

The **NOSE** is the **ONLY Organ** able to **Properly** Prepare the **Air** we **Breathe** by **Filtering, Warming** and **Beginning** the **Extraction** process of the **Breath of LIFE** in the Form of the **Oxygen NEEDED** for **LIFE**.

The **Nasal Cycle** is controlled by the **HYPOTHALAMUS**. Increased Air-flow thru the **Right Nostril** is correlated to Increased **LEFT BRAIN** Activity and **Enhanced Verbal** Performance. Increased Air-flow thru the **Left Nostril** is associated with increased **RIGHT BRAIN** Activity and **Enhanced Spatial** Performance.

The **Internal Nasal Cavities** provide 90% of the **Respiratory** System Air-Conditioning Requirements.

The **Internal Nasal Cavities** also **RECOVER** around 33% of **Exhaled HEAT** and **WATER**.

Our **Internal Temp** is a constant and consistent **98.6 Degrees**. Whenever anything is introduced in Us that is **COLDER** than our Operating Temp – our bodies have to 1st expend **ENERGY** to **Warm** it **BEFORE** it can Use it.

The **NASAL** Cavities are Created to **WARM** the **Inhaled Oxygen**, so when it reaches the **LUNGS**, no extra Energy has to be exerted = **Maximum** USE of that **Breath**.

The **Mouth** offers **NO** Warming Methods, so Large quantities of **COLD** Air gets introduced into us. This creates an environment that easily produces Dis-Eases – especially **Pneumonia** and **Asthma**. As well as numerous other **Respiratory** ailments.

Using the **Mouth** to **Inhale** can lead to the Conditions **Atelectasis** and **Emphysema** – which are basically **Poor Ventilation Micro-Areas** in the **Lungs**.

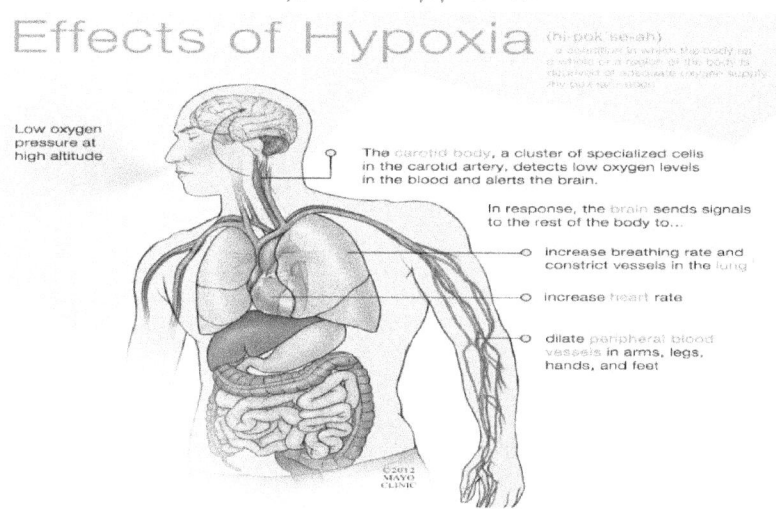

Mouth Breathing also irritates the **Tonsils** and **Adenoids**, which leads to **Tonsillitis** and **Sinus** infections, making it even harder to **Breathe** thru the **Nose**.

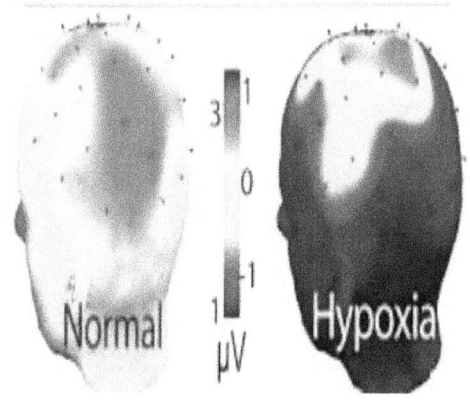

The Normal scan is from Breathing as Created – Nasal Breathing.

The Hypoxia scan is from Mouth Breathing.

Mouth Breathing is the CAUSE that creates the adverse EFFECT of Hypoxia.

OxyGen ... The Breath Of Life In Atomic Form!

Inhaling thru the **Mouth** causes **HYPER-Ventilation/HYPOXIA**. These cause a Drop BELOW normal levels of **CO2**. This **LOWERS** the amount of **Blood** and **Oxygen** to vital **Organs**, causing **Brain Hypoxia** = Fainting/Loss of Consciousness, Coma.

Hypoxic Conditions

The negative EFFECTS of Hypoxia are various and applied considerably on several Organ and Systems throughout the Body.

These are all by-products of the CAUSE of Mouth Breathing.

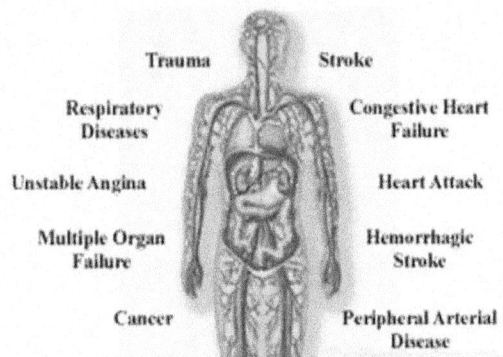

Trauma
Stroke
Respiratory Diseases
Congestive Heart Failure
Unstable Angina
Heart Attack
Multiple Organ Failure
Hemorrhagic Stroke
Cancer
Peripheral Arterial Disease

Hyper-Ventilation can only occur from using the **MOUTH** to **Breathe**. **Breathing** other-thanCreated is **The CAUSE** that produces **The EFFECT** of **DYSPNEA**. This creates a **LOW** Level of **Oxygen** IN us, which is the Environment for Dis-Eases and Cancers to grow and survive.

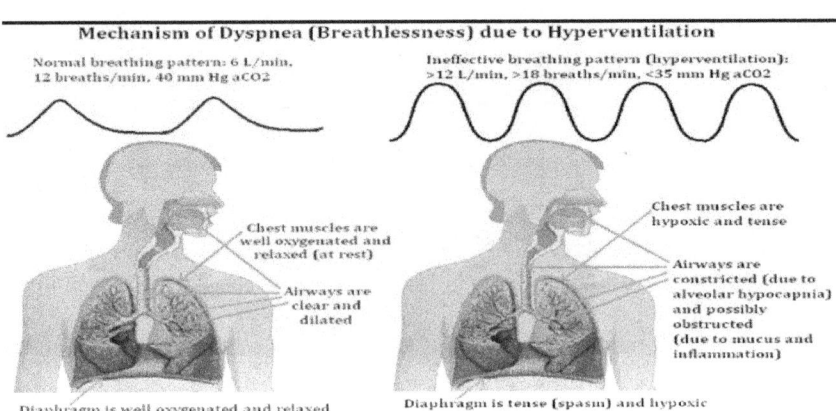

Mechanism of Dyspnea (Breathlessness) due to Hyperventilation

Normal breathing pattern: 6 L/min, 12 breaths/min, 40 mm Hg aCO2

Ineffective breathing pattern (hyperventilation): >12 L/min, >18 breaths/min, <35 mm Hg aCO2

Chest muscles are well oxygenated and relaxed (at rest)

Airways are clear and dilated

Diaphragm is well oxygenated and relaxed during exhalations and automatic pauses

Chest muscles are hypoxic and tense

Airways are constricted (due to alveolar hypocapnia) and possibly obstructed (due to mucus and inflammation)

Diaphragm is tense (spasm) and hypoxic during all phases of breathing

OxyGen ... The Breath Of Life In Atomic Form!

Whenever we **Breathe** against our Natural, **God-Created** way, we sustain almost instantaneous and irreparable damage to our **Cells**. **Oxidation** occurs from lack-of/deficient/low levels of **Oxygen**. **Oxidation** destroys the **DNA** in our **Cells**, so that when they go to Re-Generate, the create a Damaged **Cell**, that creates damaged **Tissue**, that creates damaged **Organs**, that manifests into a damaged **Us**.

REDUCTION & OXIDATION

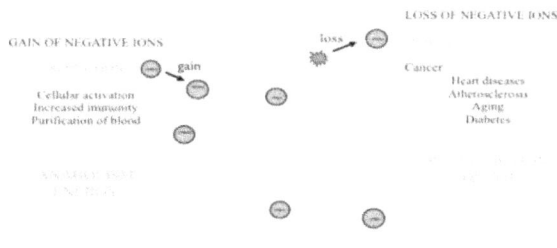

We have a Law of

Respiration. Obedience to the Law is Obedience to The **CREATOR = Abundant LIFE**.

Dis-Obedience to the Law is

Dis-Obedience to The **CREATOR** = Pre-Mature Death.

Mouth Breathing destroys the Foundation of **LIFE**.

OxyGen ... The Breath Of Life In Atomic Form!

Mouth Breathing Dis-Ease – **LONG-FACE Syndrome** = a condition developed from prolonged use of the **Mouth** to **Breathe**. It literally changes the Shape of the **Mouth** and **Face** from **Human** characteristics to those of an animal, most notably to the characteristics of a horse.

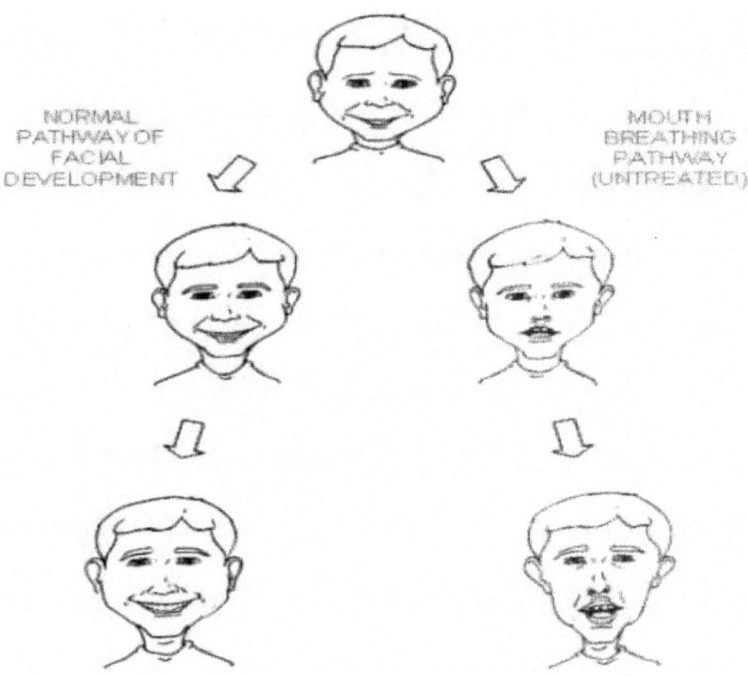

LONG FACE SYNDROME

Mouth Breathing is the **CAUSE** that produces the negative **EFFECT** of Dis-figuring of **GodCreated Beauty**. Changing ourselves from the **Image** and **Likeness** of **GOD**.

Breathing with the **Mouth** causes the Shape of the Jaw, Mouth and Teeth to become disfigured. Also, negatively affecting the Health and Condition of our **Gums**.

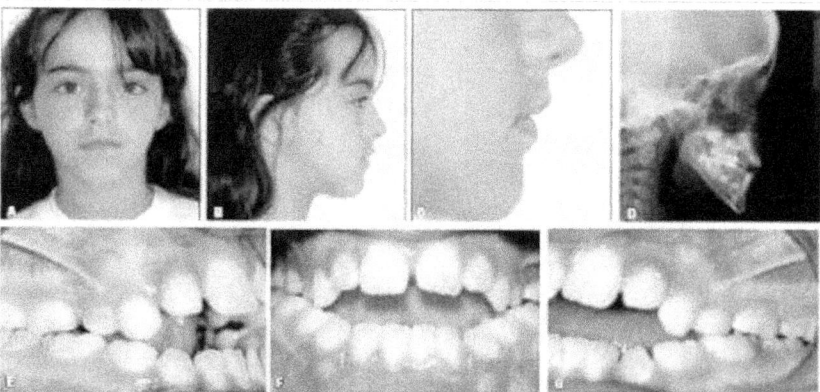

Effect of Mouth Breathing on Facial Development by Dr Mike Mew

<u>The altering of our **GOD-Created** way to Breathe **HIS** Gift of the Breath of **LIFE**, causes an Alteration in the **GOD-Created** Beauty of Us.</u>

Facial Growth and Development

Believe it or not, breathing through your mouth can actually change the shape of your face and alter your appearance. This is especially true for children because they are still growing. 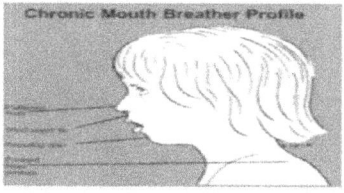 Children whose mouth breathing goes untreated may suffer from abnormal facial and dental development. Symptoms include long, narrow faces and mouths, less defined cheek bones, small lower jaws, and "weak" chins. Other facial symptoms include gummy smiles and crooked teeth. A "mouth breather" facial expression is typically not viewed as an attractive or desirable appearance to have.

WHY ASTHMA HAS BECOME AN EPIDEMIC :

Human hair is the dominant particle of pollutants in the air. Pet dander, Mold spores, dust mite and several other particles are

SWALLOWED when one

Inhales thru the **Mouth**.

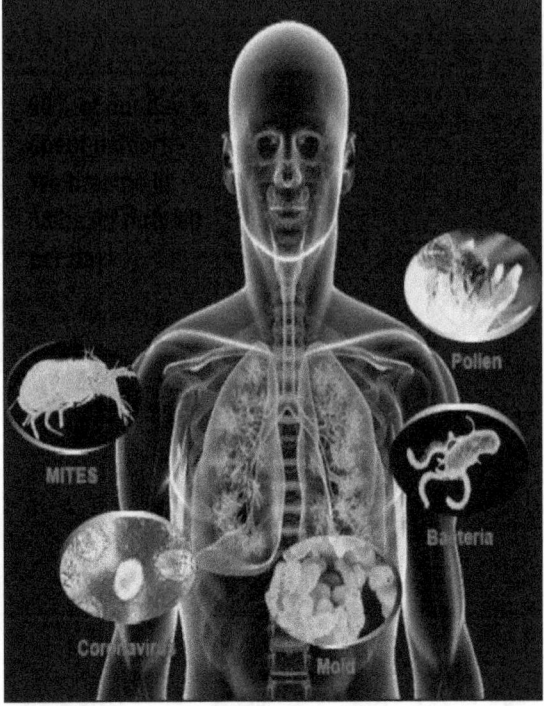

From Natural elements to man-made pollutants, we when **Inhale,** we take in more than **Oxygen**. The **Nose** is our Natural defense against these Pollutants.

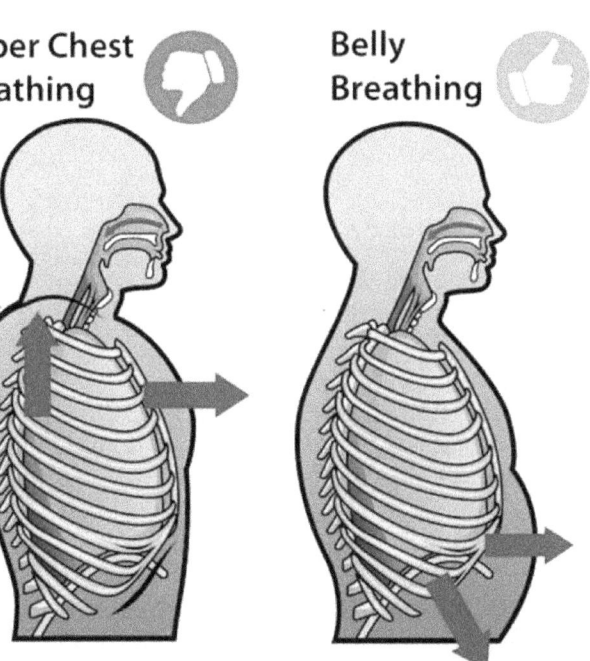

OxyGen ... The Breath Of Life In Atomic Form!

Chapter 10 ...... Nasal vs Mouth Exhalation

*****

The Process of **Exhaling** is also referred to as **Expiration**.

Just as the **Nose** was Created to Inhale the **Breath Of LIFE**, it is also our Primary Exit.

The process of **Exhaling** is just as vital as **Inhaling**, with it's own adverse conditions when performed other-than Created = with the **Mouth**.

A FULL and Purposeful **Exhaling** helps clear-out the **Lungs**, so that we can take-in a Fuller **InBreath** that provides Fresh **Oxygenated Air**.

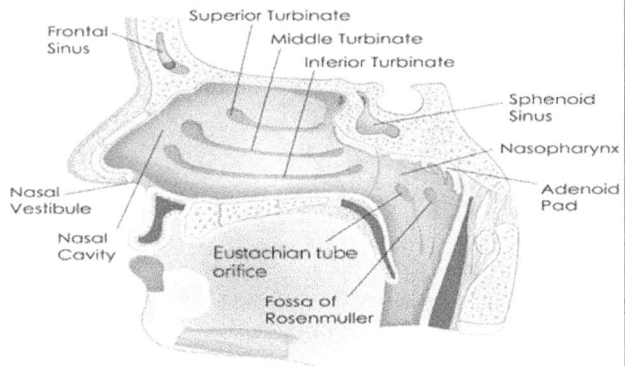

The **Nasal** Cavities and

Passages are Perfectly

Created to prepare the **Breath** Of **Life** for use.

Knowing and understanding the anatomy of the **Nose** allows one to Maximize the **Energy** of **Oxygen**.

OxyGen ... The Breath Of Life In Atomic Form!

The **Internal Nose** provides **90%** of the **Respirator** Air-Conditioning requirements and recovers approximately **33%** of Exhaled **Heat** and **Moisture**.

The **Absorption** and **Extraction** of **Oxygen** occurs primarily during **Exhale**.

The **Nostrils** are **Smaller**, so **Exhaling** thru them creates a **Slower Exhalation** and Builds up Greater **Air Pressure**. These conditions give the **Lungs** extra **Time** to **Extract** a greater amount of **Oxygen** = producing the Proper amount of **Oxygen** to Perform **Maximum Cellular Respiration**.

Exhaling thru the **Mouth** causes the Brain to **'THINK'** that too much **Carbon Dioxide** is escaping too fast. So, the **Brain** becomes stimulated and begins to activate the production of **Mucous** – Causing **Excess Mucous Build-Up**.

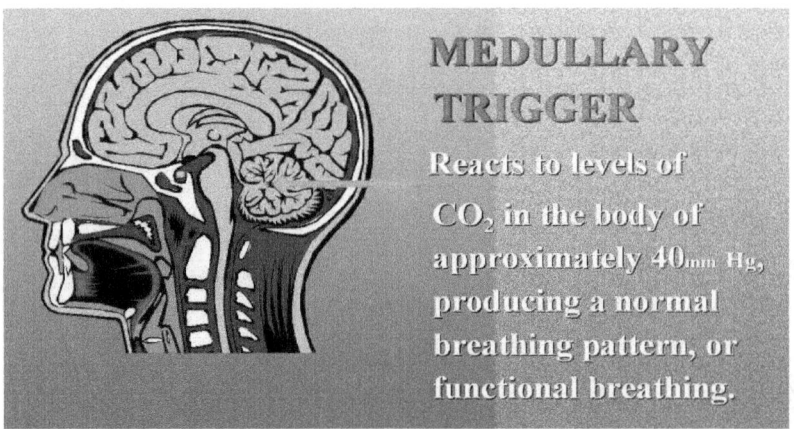

MEDULLARY TRIGGER
Reacts to levels of CO_2 in the body of approximately 40mm Hg, producing a normal breathing pattern, or functional breathing.

Proper **Oxygen** - **Carbon Dioxide** exchange maintains the **Blood PH** (Potential/Power of Hydrogen). If **Carbon Dioxide** is lost too quickly (as with **Mouth Breathing**) = **Oxygen** absorption is **Decreased** = **Lowered PH** Level = ability to become Sick, ill, dis-eased.

Mouth breathing can cause a dangerously excessive build-up of **CO2** in our bodies. **Oxygen** is absorbed on the **Exhale** and the backpressure created from Properly **Exhaling** through the **Nose** allows for maximum transfer and exchange of **Oxygen** and **Carbon Dioxide**.

Mouth breathing lacks the backpressure so there is less **Oxygen** and **Carbon Dioxide** transferred and exchanged = increase to Dangerous levels of **CO2** in Self.

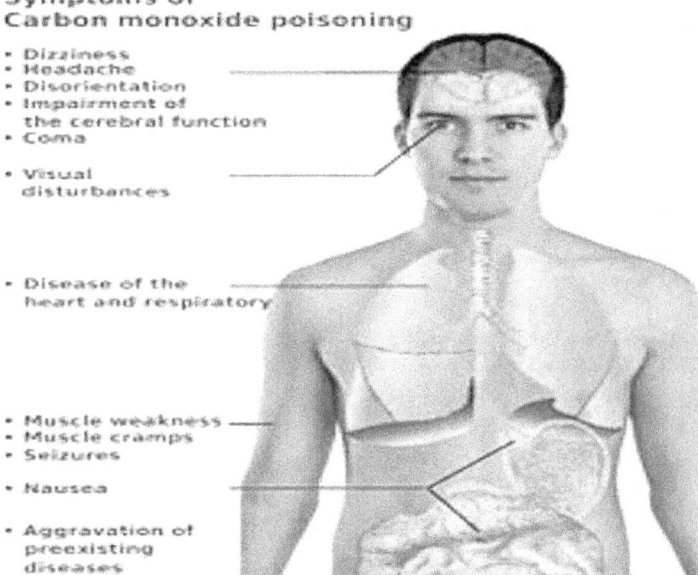

Symptoms of Carbon monoxide poisoning

- Dizziness
- Headache
- Disorientation
- Impairment of the cerebral function
- Coma
- Visual disturbances
- Disease of the heart and respiratory
- Muscle weakness
- Muscle cramps
- Seizures
- Nausea
- Aggravation of preexisting diseases

Each **Nostril** is innervated by **5 Cranial Nerves** from a different side of the Brain. Each **Nostril** functions independently and synergistically in **Filtering, Warming, Dehumidifying** and **Smelling** the **Air**. Using the **Mouth**, offers NO form of Filtering, Warming or Dehumidifying abilities = Polluted and Cold Air that damages the **Lungs** and creates detrimental conditions.

Nasal Breathing imposes approximately **50%** More Resistance to the **Air** stream than **Mouth Breathing** does – resulting in **10-20%** More **Oxygen** Up-take.

Afferent Stimuli from the **Nerves** that Regulate **Breathing** are in the **Nasal Passages**. The Inhaled **Air** passes thru the **Nasal Mucosa** and carries the **Stimuli** to the **Reflex Nerves** that control **Breathing**. Mouth Breathing by-passes the **Nasal Mucosa** – making Regular **Breathing** harder.

Focused and Strong **Exhalation** strengthens the **Chest** and **Abdomen Muscles**. And gives us more control over our **Breathing** = Reducing shortness of **Breath** and other **Breathing** conditions.

OxyGen ... The Breath Of Life In Atomic Form!

TEETH GRINDING AND LOW OXYGEN LEVELS

With teeth grinding being the most obvious form of abnormal jaw movement due to the noise made as the teeth clash against each other, there are also subtle jaw movements that we can measure.

Interestingly, these small movements seem to relate to intermittent low oxygen levels.

Dumais IE et al. J Oral Rehabil. 2015 Jul 1.

> Could transient hypoxia be associated with rhythmic masticatory muscle activity in sleep bruxism in the absence of sleep-disordered breathing? A preliminary report.

Teeth grinding also seems to tie in with changes in blood pressure. We will come back to mentioning blood pressure later on.

Nashed A et al. Sleep. 2012 Apr 1;35(4):529-36.

> Sleep bruxism is associated with a rise in arterial blood pressure.

Proper **Exhalation** helps **Reduce Stress** and *Lowers* **Blood Pressure** by stimulating the Calming **Parasympathetic Nervous System**. Using the **Mouth** exacerbates **Stress** and Increases **Blood Pressure**.

Our **Nose** makes approximately **2 Pints** of **Mucous** everyday. Excessive **Mucous** build-up is the root cause of a majority of the sicknesses and diseases that we suffer from. Improper breathing creates a potentially dangerous and detrimental build-up of it.

Benefits of Deeper breathing... physical

- Increased purification of blood
- Decrease in Toxins
- Increase Digestion
- Decrease Waste
- Improved Nervous System
- Improves functioning the glands, producing chemical requirements of the body
- Improves Lungs capacity & resistance
- Reduces Heart load & makes Heart live longer
- Controls Weight of the body
- Regulate Heat & cooling System of the body
- Improves Health & reduces weakness
- Oxygen to brain & mind relaxes

OxyGen ... The Breath Of Life In Atomic Form!

Chapter 11 ...... OxyGen and the Brain

*****

Oxygen is the Most Important ingredient for the growth and development of a fully functional **Brain** that can operate at its maximum potential – which is **_LIMITLESS_** !!!

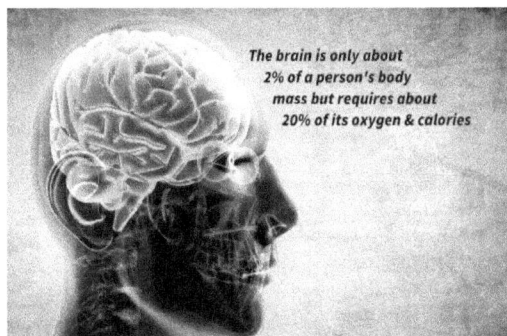

The brain is only about 2% of a person's body mass but requires about 20% of its oxygen & calories

Despite it's small **Tissue Mass**, the important role of the **Brain** requires the most **Oxygen** per **Tissue**/Body part.

The **Brain** manifests the **Breath**

Of **Life** into the **Electrical Energy** needed for Life Functions.

Food/nutrition and **Hydration**/water are the remaining necessary components for a healthy brain, but without **Oxygen,** one is scientifically and medically diagnosed as Brain-dead.

When we **Breathe**, **Eat**, **Drink** according our anatomical function and stay physically active, we create the proper environment for successfully achieving and maintaining Supreme Health and Fitness !

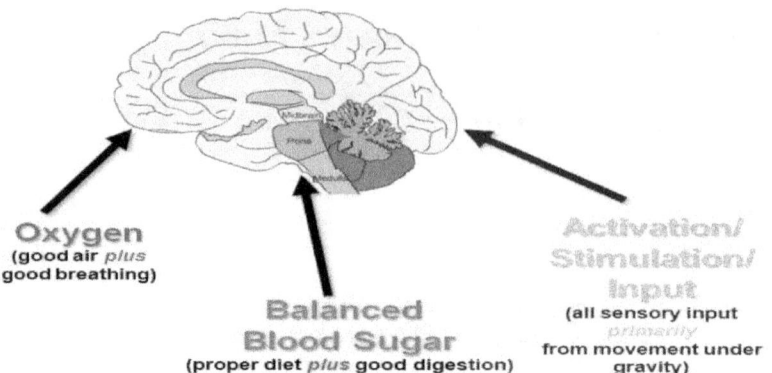

Once we fall below **96%** we are **Oxygen** deficient and suffer from the effects of lack of **Oxygen**. Normal **Brain** functions ad activities are severely impaired. Producing and maintaining high quality **Thoughts** become difficult.

Our **Brains** need a steady of **Oxygen** to be considered healthy.

Normal body functions require more **Energy** and effort to achieve and maintain **Homeostasis**. After a prolonged state of **Oxygen** deprivation, the manifestation of **Brain** defects become diagnosed and pronounced. With the potential of causing pre-mature death.

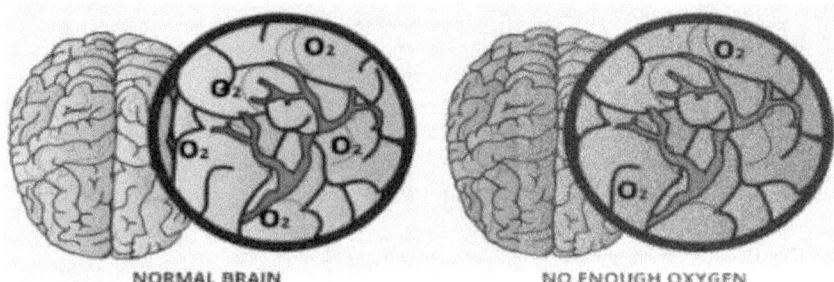

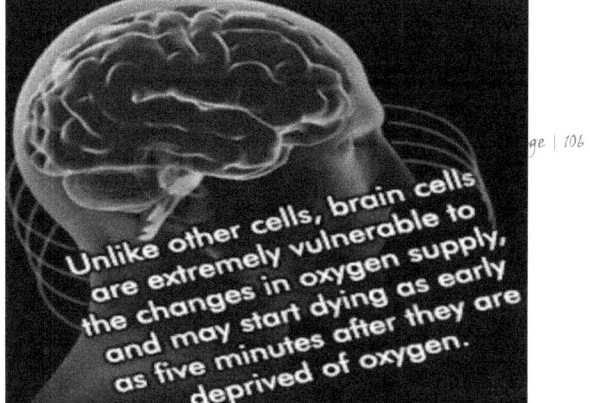

Brain Cells start to decrease in function and die when the body becomes Oxygen deficient. The damage increases the longer one remains Oxygen deficient.

Strokes, also called a 'Brain Attack', is the sudden death of **Brain Cells** due to lack of **Oxygen** and occurs when the **Blood** supply to the **Brain** is interrupted and/of severely reduced which deprives the **Brain Tissues** of **Oxygen** and **Nutrients**.

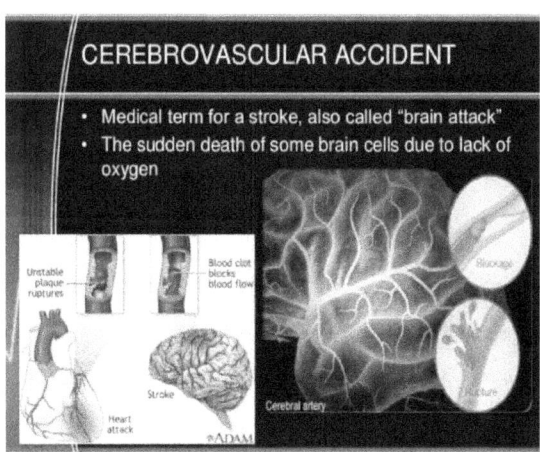

Lack of **Oxygen** is an easy condition to produce. After **ONE** minute of the use of the **Mouth** for **Respiration** creates the Lack of **Oxygen** that destroys **Brain**. Every 5 to 10 minutes of improper breathing exacerbates the depth of **Brain** dysfunction and death.

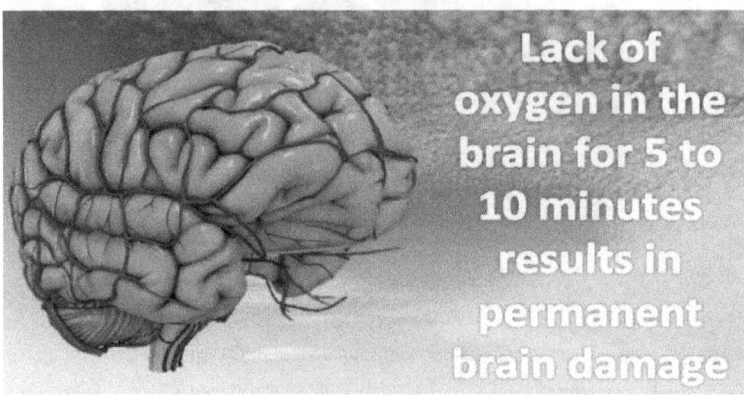

A majority of the population suffers small, barely noticed **Strokes** that occurs throughout their state of deficiency. **Mental Clarity**, **Recall**, **Focus** and **Power** are all **Oxygen** dependent.

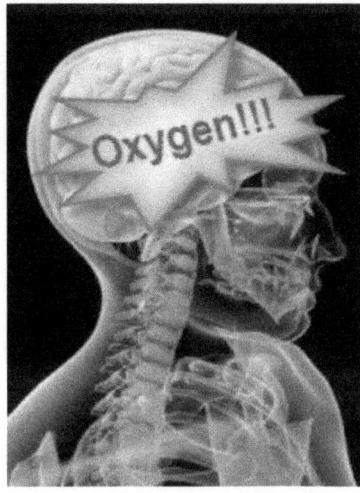

Symptoms Of An Oxygen Deprived Brain

Neurons in oxygen deprived brains begin to misfire and can take a toll on mental and emotional health. It has been estimated that a healthy brain has 35,000 thoughts per day. Of these, 96% are repetitive or useless. Some simple math tells us that we only have about 1,400 useful thoughts per day. On the other hand, an oxygen deprived brain has about 85,000 thoughts per day!

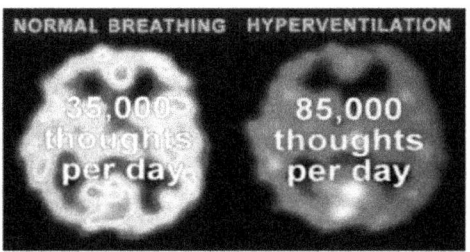

If we assume that an oxygen deprived brain still has 1,400 useful thoughts per day, that means a brain starved for oxygen has an additional 50,000 useless or repetitive thoughts in a day-enough to drive anyone crazy! This is mental clutter. Some manifestations of oxygen deprivation to the brain include:

- *Rehashing a mistake or a bad experience* – The past is in the past. It can't be changed. **But a brain starved for oxygen enjoys replaying every detail of every bad experience.** Constantly leaving us wondering what we could have done differently...or more likely, what the other person could have done differently.

- *Inventing terrifying and highly unlikely scenarios* – As the neurons keep misfiring, our imagination goes into overdrive. **We begin imagining horrifying outcomes to the everyday decisions that we make.** We are suddenly terrified that if today's presentation at work doesn't go perfectly, we are going to get fired, lose our house, lose our spouse, and end up living alone in a van down by the river.

- *Uncontrollable emotions* – As these tens of thousands of useless thoughts go through our heads, **they take us on an emotional roller coaster.** We are up...and then we are down. We can't be reasoned with. We often feel like the world is crashing in around us. We find ourselves overreacting to even the tiniest of offenses. We can't justify the way we feel...because it doesn't make sense.

OxyGen ... The Breath Of Life In Atomic Form!

Chapter 12 ... Oxidation & Oxidative Stress/Damage

*****

When **Cells** use **Oxygen** to generate **Energy**, **Free-radicals** are created from the formation of **Adenosine Triphosphate (ATP)** in the **Mitochondria**.

This process is also known as **Oxidation/Oxidative** Stress.

> **Oxidation Definition:** Oxidation is the loss of electrons during a reaction by a molecule, atom or ion.
>
> Oxidation occurs when the oxidation state of a molecule, atom or ion is increased.
>
> An older meaning of oxidation was when oxygen was added to a compound. Example: Iron combines with oxygen to form iron oxide or rust. The iron is said to have oxidized into rust.

Oxidation is the **Natural** byproduct of the normal **Metabolism** of **Oxygen**. This Metabolizing process produces **REACTIVE OXYGEN SPECIES (ROS)** and **REACTIVE NITROGEN SPECIES (RNS)**.

Because of their close association with **Cellular Respiration**, **ROS** and **RNS** are usually termed together.

ROS/RNS play a dual role. They are both **Beneficial** and **Toxic** compounds.

OxyGen ... The Breath Of Life In Atomic Form!

At Low/Moderate levels, **ROS/RNS** exert Beneficial effects on **Cellular** responses and **Immune** function. At **HIGH** concentrations, they generate **OXIDATIVE** Stress.

Oxidative Stress plays a Major part in the development of chronic and degenerative ailments.

ROS/RNS are the terms used to collectively describe **Free-Radicals** and other **Non-Radical Reactive Derivatives** – also called **OXIDANTS**.

Greatest enemy to our health is free radicals

FORMATION of **ROS/RNS** can occur in our **Cells** by 2 ways = **ENZYMATIC** and **NON-ENZYMATIC** Reactions.

ENZYMATIC Reactions that generate **Free-radicals**, are formulated from the **Respiratory** Chain. **NON-ENZYMATIC** Reactions are generated from Outside influences – Pollutants, Smoke, Emotional/Mental/Spiritual Stress.

GENERATION of **ROS/RNS** can occur from **Endogenous** and **Exogenous** sources.

Endogenous ROS/RNS Oxidants are formed from **Immune Cell** activation, Inflammation, Exercise, Mental/Emotional/Spiritual Stress, infections.

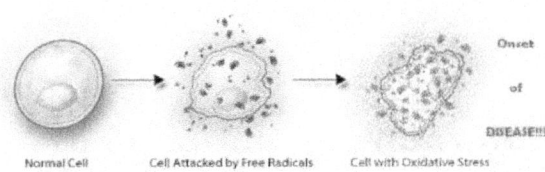

Reactive oxygen species (• unpaired electrons)

Oxygen	Superoxide anion	Peroxide	Hydroxyl radical	Hydroxyl ion
O_2	$O_2^{\bullet -}$	$O_2^{\bullet -2}$	$\cdot OH$	OH^-

Exogenous ROS/RNS Oxidants result from Air and Water pollution, smoke, alcohol, smoked/cooked Meats, industrial cleaners, heavy/transition metals and radiation. After penetration **INTO** our Bodies, these Exogenous compounds are metabolized/decomposed into **Free-Radicals**.

For our **Biological** System, **ROS** Oxidants are the main focus.

ROS are chemically active **Molecules** containing **Oxygen**. **ROS** have important roles in **Cell Signaling** and **Homeostasis**.

The term **ROS** encompasses all highly-reactive, **Oxygen**-containing **Molecules**, including **FreeRadicals**.

Types of **ROS** include the **Hydroxyl Radical**, **Hydrogen Peroxide**, the **Superoxide Anion Radical**, **Nitric Oxide Radical** and various **Lipid Peroxides**. These **ROS** can react (pos/neg) with the **Membrane Lipids**, **Nucleic Acids**, **Proteins**, **Enzymes** and other small **Molecules** of our **Cells**.

During times of **Environmental** Stress (**UV** or **HEAT** exposure), **Exogenous** Sources (**Ionizing Radiation, Pollutants, Drugs, Cigarette** Smoke) or **Emotional** Stress (**Anger, Worry, Arousal**) the **ROS Levels** can **INCREASE**. An Increase in **ROS** levels then becomes **Damaging** to **Cell Growth** and **Development**.

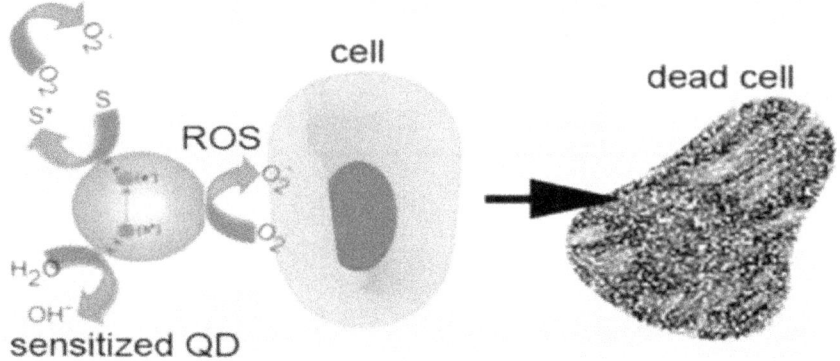

<u>This Increase in ROS is known as OXIDATIVE STRESS = the DEATH of a Cell !</u>

OxyGen ... The Breath Of Life In Atomic Form!

Using the **Mouth** to **Breathe Increases** the **Harmful Effects** of the **Natural** occurring **ROS**. **ROS** in this state can damage **DNA**, **RNA** and **Proteins** = the **Physiology** of **Aging** (Alzheimer's and other age-related decline Brain functioning).

RNS are a family of **Anti-Microbial Molecules** derived from **Nitric Oxide (-NO2)** and **Superoxide (O2-)** that are produced via **Enzymatic**-activity of inducible **Nitric Oxide Synthase 2 (NOS2)** and **NADPH Oxidase**.

Physiology	Consequence/function:	Pathophysiology

ROS/RNS involvement in physiological processes	ROS/RNS involvement in pathophysiological processes
Regulation of vascular tone	Age related diseases (aging)
Regulation of cell adhesion	Malignant transformation
Amplification of immune response	Atherosclerosis
Programmed cells death	Neurodegenerative disease
Receptor mediated signaling pathways	Rheumatoid arthritis
	Ischemia reperfusion injury
	Obstructive sleep apnea
	Obesity and diabetes

RNS act together with **ROS** to damage **Cells**, causing **Nitrosative Stress**.

RNS are continuously produced in **Plants** as by-products of **Aerobic Metabolism** or in response to **stress**.

RNS is produced in us with the reaction of **Nitric Oxide (-NO)** with **Superoxide (O2-)** To form **Peroxynitrite (ONOO-)**.

OxyGen ... The Breath Of Life In Atomic Form!

This is important because **Nitric Oxide** is a **KEY** mediator in main **Bodily** functions including **Regulation** of **Smooth Muscle Tone** and **Blood Pressure**, **Platelet Activation** and **Vascular Cell Signaling**.

Oxidation is the Normal byproduct of **Breathing**. This **Oxidative** state causes the **ROS** to increase the Decline of **Aging** by negatively affecting the **Efficiency** of **Mitochondria** = further Increasing the Rate of **ROS** production.

Causes of Oxidative Stress

Oxidation is a Natural occurring reaction to Life.
Inhaling the Breath Of Life as Created is the catalyst to creating our Natural Anti-Oxidants

OXIDATIVE STRESS!

Causes shown:
- Smoking
- Diet
- Medication & Treatments
- Air & Water Pollutants
- Fast Foods [McDonald's]
- Stress
- Lack of Good Nutrition
- Inadequate amounts of physical activity
- Alcohol
- Pesticides
- Exposure to Toxins
- Inadequate Intake of Fruits & Vegetables
- Contaminants
- Excessive Exercise

Just about everything we do results in oxidation (or inflammation) producing potentially damaging free radicals!

Oxidative Stress means an In-Balance between **Pro-Oxidant** and **Anti-Oxidant Mechanisms**. This results in excessive **Oxidative** Metabolism. This Stress can be due to several environmental factors such as – Poor Diet, Medications, Pollutants, Radiation, Toxins, etc.

This can cause **Oxidative** damage to our **Cells DNA**, **Proteins** and other **Macro-Molecules** that lead to a wide-range of Human Dis-eases – most notably – **HEART DIS-EASE** and **CANCER**. Both of these health conditions are the leading Causes of Pre-Mature DEATH!!

OxyGen ... The Breath Of Life In Atomic Form!

Chapter 13 ... Respiration & Cellular Respiration

*****

Respiration is the act of **Breathing**/gathering in the necessary amount of **Oxygen** to supply the **Cells** with the **Energy** to break-down food for **Energy**.

Respiration is also know as **Energy Transfer Reaction**. Every **Organism** uses the **Chemical** process of **Respiration** to transfer **Energy** into a **Usable Chemical** (**ATP**) Form.

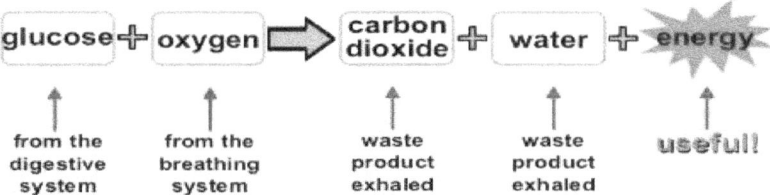

Transferring of stored **Chemical Energy** in food to a form of **Energy** we can use requires the exchange of **Oxygen** between an **Organism** and it's **Environment**.

Respiration is a continual process in the **Cells** of all **Living** forms.

Respiration occurs in the **Mitochondria** in our **Cells**. All **Cells** contain **Mitochondria**, but can contain different amounts.

Muscle Cells and some Organs and Tissues carry-out lots of Respiration, so they contain large amounts of Mitochondria. They have Thin-walls to allow substances to pass thru. They have large surface Cells to allow many Reactions to take place at once.

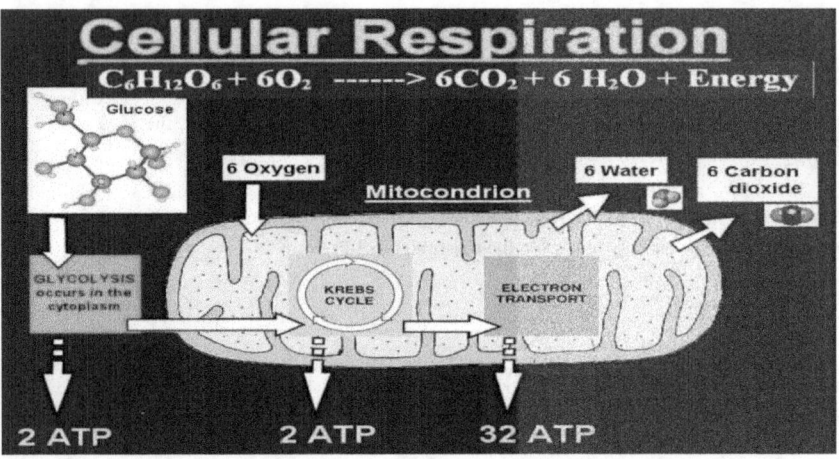

*Elements for Respiration include = 1. Glucose, 2. Oxygen, 3. Enzymes mix the ingredients in the Mitochondria and produce ATP. CO2 an H2O are the waste by-products of Respiration.

*Chemical Equation for Respiration = C6, H12, O6 + O2 Enzymes H2O + CO2 + 36 ATP's.

*Word Equation for Respiration = Glucose + Oxygen = Water + Carbon Dioxide + Energy.

The ATP gained from Respiration is easily Hydrolyzed = Energy is released and ADP is formed.

$$ATP + H2 = ADP + P + Energy.$$

Respiration is a series of actions in which Energy is released from Glucose.

OxyGen ... The Breath Of Life In Atomic Form!

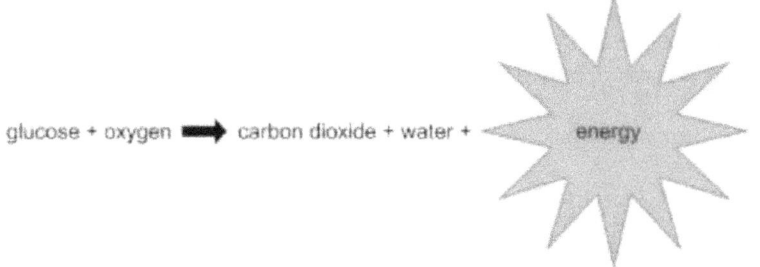

Glucose is a **Sugar** from **Food** which the **Body** uses in the **Cells** to make **Energy** in **Respiration**.

Respiration - Glucose + Oxygen - Carbon Dioxide + Water + Energy Transfer.

Cellular Respiration is the **Release** of **Energy** from **Foods**. **Cell Respiration** requires an adequate/precise amount of **Oxygen** to properly process foods into **Energy**.

Important **Cellular Respiration** is the **Enzyme**-controlled **Reactions** in which **Energy** of **Food** (**Glucose**) is converted into an usable form of **Energy** = **ATP**. All **Cells** function on the **Energy** Released from **ATP** and carry out **ALL LIFE** functions using **ATP Energy**.

Cellular Respiration is the ENERGY for LIFE. It is the set of **3 Main Metabolic** reactions and processes that take place in our **Cells** to convert **Bio-Chemical** (**Atomic**) **Energy** from

Nutrients, like GLUCOSE and convert it into the **Atomic Elements - Carbon Dioxide** (CO_2) and **Water** (H_2O). This is ATOMIC Conversion.

The **Atomic Energy** that's released is converted into the **Bio-Chemical** form of **ADENOSINE TRIPHOSPHATE** (**ATP**). **ATP** is used for **ALL** Energy-consuming activities of the **Cell** = **Cellular Growth** & **Development**. This is the 2nd **Metabolic Reaction**.

The 3rd **Metabolic Reaction** involves the **Atomic Waste** = **Free-Radicals**. Naturally forming **Free-Radicals** from the Conversions and Use of the **Atoms** of Foods we eat.

ATP is Hydrolyzed Energy. The **Mitochondria** in our **Cells** have **Enzymes** that use **Oxygen** to get the **Energy OUT** of **Food** – also called **AEROBIC Cellular Respiration**.

OxyGen ... The Breath Of Life In Atomic Form!

Cellular Respiration is dependent upon an **Aerobic** (**Oxygen**) Environment.

Cellular Respiration uses **3** conversions to break-down **Glucluse** into its lowest **Atomic** denominator. The Process **GLYCOLYSIS** (splitting of Sugar) occurs **1st** by converting **Glucose** from **Chemical** form and into **PYRUVIC ACID**.

The **Pyruvic Acid** is broken down into **Molecular** Form - in the **Molecule** of **ACETYL COA**.

In the presence of **Oxygen** (O_2) Gas, all the **Hydrogens** (H_2) are stripped off the **Acetyl CoA** to Extract the **Electrons** for Creating **ATP** (**Energy**).

All that remains of the **Sugar/Glucose** is the **WASTE** - Carbon Dioxide (CO_2) and H_2O (**EXHALE/Water**) to be **Exhaled OUT**.

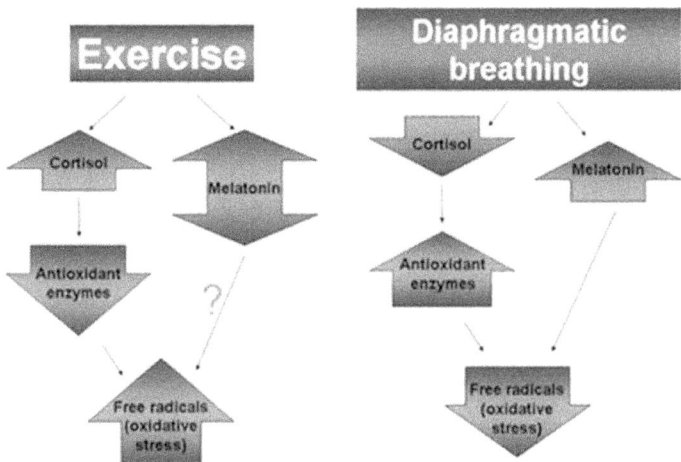

Chapter 14 ... OxyGen – Cell Hypoxia - Free-Radicals - Cancer

*****

The Natural occurring result creating **Energy** thru **Cellular Respiration**, is responsible for the creation of **FREE-RADICALS**. <u>LOW</u> **Energy**, Easy-to-Neutralize Free-Radicals.

Free-Radicals are un-stable **Atoms** that are missing an **Electron** in its Outer-ring of **Electrons**. To be **STABLE**, an **Atoms** Outer-ring of **Electrons MUST** be **EVEN**.

ANTI-OXIDANTS are the Natural trigger to **STOP** the Natural occurring **Free-Radical Atom**.

Cell Hypoxia is the Main **CAUSE** of **HIGH Energy/Hard-to-Neutralize**, **Free-Radical** generation and **Oxidative Stress** – The **EFFECT**.

Improper **Breathing** (**Mouth / Chest**) causes a **LOW Body Oxygen Level** – making **Cells Hypoxic**. This means that they switch to **ANAEROBIC** (without **Oxygen**) **Respiration** and to start producing **Lactic Acid** and other **In-Completely Oxidized Chemicals** or **Free-Radicals** = **Cellular** Stress = **Oxidation** = Sicknesses, Dis-Eases and Pre-Mature DEATH.

Mouth/Chest Breathing creates Less-than Normal **Carbon Dioxide** (CO_2) Levels, causing a condition referred to as **Arterial Hypercapnia** (CO_2 Deficiency). **Arterial Hypercapnia** causes **Tissue Hypoxia**.

Cell Oxygen Levels are controlled by **Alveolar Carbon Dioxide** (CO_2) and Proper **Breathing**

(**Nose / Diaphragm**). Hyperventilation, regardless of **Arterial CO_2** changes, causes **Alveolar Hypercapnia** – which leads to **Cell Hypoxia** (**LOW Cell Oxygen** concentrations.

Hyperventilation Decreases **Body Oxygenation** that leads to **Hypocapnia Vasoconstriction** of **Blood Vessels** – LESS **Oxygen** released by **Red Blood Cells** – Inadequate **Blood** supply to Main **Organs** (**Brain** being 1st as it takes **20%** 0f **Oxygen** per **Breath**).

The CAUSE of Not **Breathing** as Created, produces **The EFFECT** of Diminished **Brain Function** = Easily Led in the **Wrong** Direction …. Hard to Lead to the **RIGHT** !

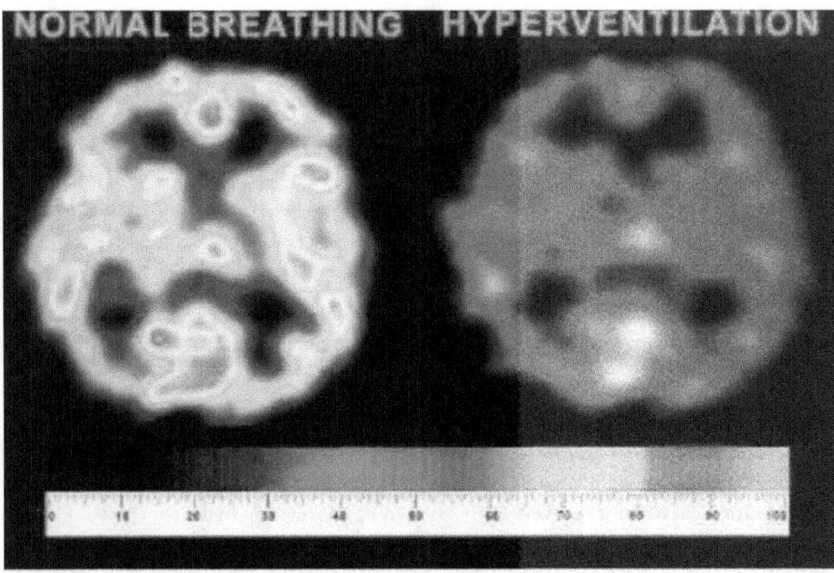

Effects of 1 minute of voluntary hyperventilation on brain oxygen levels (vasoconstriction due to a lack of CO2)

Hyperventilation, **Hypoxia** and **Hypercapnia** can ONLY be caused by **MOUTH Breathing**.

When a **Free-Radical Atom** is created, it seeks to re-gain its missing **Electron** from the Closet **STABLE Atom**... This in-turns makes that once **Stable Atom**, turn into a **Free-Radical**....REPEATING the process.

If these **Free-Radical Atoms** aren't stopped – they develop into **Molecules** that develop into **Tissues** that develop into **Tumors** that Negatively affect surrounding **Organs/Bones** = **CANCER** !

Cancer has only **ONE Primary** cause = the **REPLACEMENT** of **Normal Oxygen Respiration** of the body's **Cells** by an **Oxygen Deficient Cell Respiration**.

MANY scientist believe that a consistent **LOW-Level/LACK** of **Oxygen MUST** be held responsible for the **FORMATION & FURTHERANCE** of **Cancer Cells**, thus being one of the **Causes** of **CANCER** !!

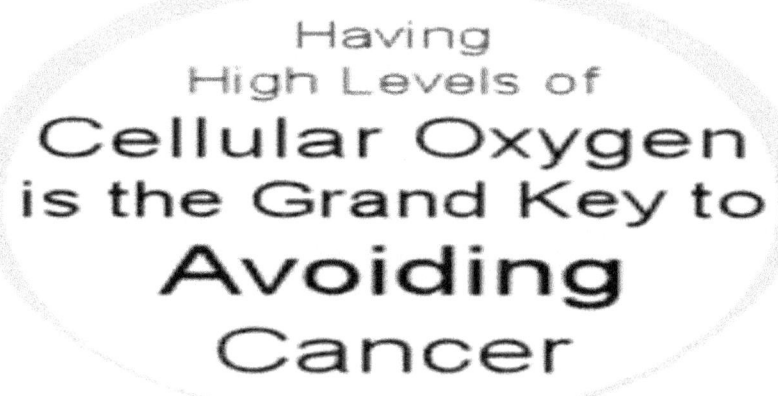

A **DEFICIENT** and **INSUFFICIENT** supply of **Oxygen** to the **TISSUES** is linked with such conditions as **HEART DISEASE, ANAEMIA, ACUTE POISONINGS**, and Many other Detrimental Issues.

Within **ALL** Serious Diseases – **LOW Oxygen Levels** are Always Apparent….**HYPOXIA** – Lack of **Oxygen** in the **Cells/Tissues** is the Fundamental Cause for **ALL Degenerative** Issues !!!

Low Oxygen levels create **ROS**. **ROS** are constantly generated and eliminated in our **Biological** system. **ROS** are required to drive regulatory pathways.

Under normal **Physiologic** conditions, **Cells** are able to Control **ROS** levels by Balancing the Generation of **ROS** with their Elimination. However, under **OXIDATIVE** Stress conditions, these **ROS** damage **Cellular Proteins**, **Lipids** and **DNA**, causing **Lesions** in **Cells** that contribute to **CARCINOGENESIS**.

Cancer Cells exhibit greater **ROS** Stress than normal **Cells**. This is due to increased **Metabolic** activity and **Mitochondrial Malfunction**.

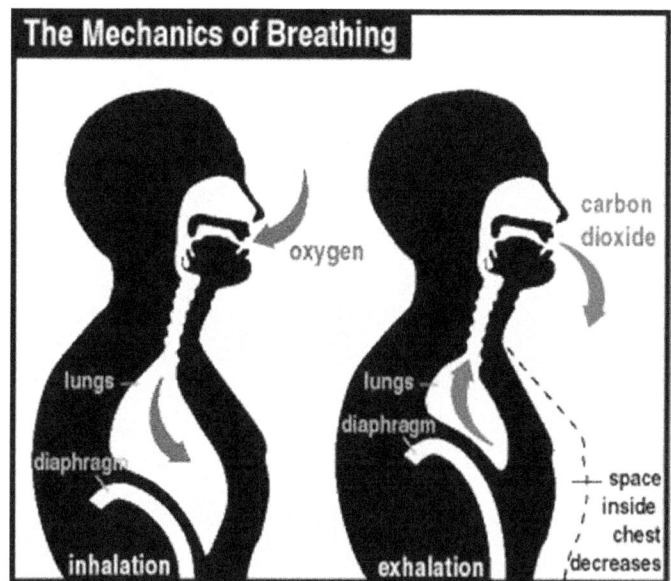

OxyGen ... The Breath Of Life In Atomic Form!

Chapter 15 ... OxyGen & Anti-Oxidants

*****

Just as the **Natural** process of **Cellular Respiration** generates **Low-Energy** (**Less Damaging / Easily Neutralized**) **Free-Radicals**, we are Created with **Bodies** that have several **Natural** mechanisms to counter-act **Oxidative** stress by producing **Anti-Oxidants**, naturally generated '**In Situ'** (**Endogenous Anti-Oxidants**) or have them **Externally** supplied thru **Foods** (**Exogenous Anti-Oxidants**).

The role of these **Anti-Oxidants** are to **NEUTRALIZE** the excess of **Free-Radicals**, to **Protect** the **Cells** against their **Toxic** effects and to **Contribute** to **Dis-Ease Prevention**.

The **Breath of LIFE - Oxygen (O2)** and **Carbon Dioxide (O2)** are the **BEST** NATURAL ANTIOXIDANTS. **THE CREATOR** gave us a Ever-Perfecting, Self-Maintaining, Long-Lasting Vehicle to **Express** the **Spirit** of **HIMSELF** that's **IN US**.

ALL WE HAVE TO DO IS FOLLOW THE LAWS THAT GOVERN SELF !!!

Endogenous compounds in our **Cells** can be classified as **Enzymatic** and **Non-Enzymatic AntiOxidants**.

The **Anti-Oxidant Enzymes - GLUTATHIONE PEROXIDASE (GPx), CATALASE (CAT), GLUTATHIONE REDUCTASE (GRx)** and **SUPEROXIDE DISMUTASE (SOD)** are **Naturally** Produced by our **Bodies** to stop the Natural effects **Cellular Respiration**.

$$O_2^{\cdot -} + O_2^{\cdot -} \xrightarrow{\text{SOD}} O_2 + H_2O_2$$

Superoxide Dismutase is our **1st** Line of **Defense** against **Free-Radicals**. SOD catalyzes the Conversion of the **Superoxide Anion Radical** (a strong damaging radical) INTO **Hydrogen Peroxide (H2O2)** (a milder radical) and **Oxygen (O2)** by Reduction.

The **Oxidant** formed into **H2O2** is further **Neutralized** and converted into **Water (H2O)** and **Oxygen (O2)** by the Enzyme **Catalase (CAT)** and/or **Glutathione Peroxidase (GPx)**.

Glutathione Peroxidase are **Enzymes** that are similar to **Catalase**, in which they help degrade **Hydrogen Peroxide**. The also reduce Organic **Peroxides** into **Alcohol** – allowing further avenue for the Elimination of Toxic Oxidants.

These **Enzymes** *REQUIRE* **Micro-Nutrients** co-factors for their **Activation**. These **MicroNutrients** are derived from our **Foods**.

The **Importance** of Practicing *HOW TO EAT TO LIVE !!!*

These **Micro-Nutrients** include : SELENIUM, IRON, COPPER, ZINC and MANGANESE.

SOD's are Metal-containing **Enzymes** that Depend on a bond of **Copper**, **Iron** or **Zinc** to activate their **Anti-Oxidant** properties.

All of these Anti-Oxidants ACTIVATORS are found in the Wonderful Small, White NAVY BEAN!!

Besides the Enzymatic **Anti-Oxidants** that are Naturally Produced by our **Bodies**, we have a wide-variety of **Foods** that are available for their **Anti-Oxidant Nutrient** properties.

There are **4 Non-Enzymatic Anti-Oxidants** that play a major role in the **Protection** of our **Cells**. They are VITAMIN C, VITAMIN E, GLUTATHIONE and BETA CAROTENE

*VITAMIN C – the most Important **Water-Soluble Anti-Oxidant** in **Extracellular Fluids**. **Vitamin C** helps to Neutralize **ROS** in the Water/Aqueous phase – **BEFORE** it can Attack our **Cellular LIPIDS.**

*VITAMIN E – is the most Important **Lipid Soluble Anti-Oxidant.**

Vitamin E is important as a Chain-breaking **Anti-Oxidant** within the **Cell Membrane**. It can Protect the **Membrane Fatty-Acids** from **Lipid Peroxidation**.

Vitamin E's major role is to trap **Peroxy Radical's** in **Cellular Membranes**.

VITAMIN E BECOMES A FREE-RADICAL, BUT IS REGENERATED BY VITAMIN C !! *** GLUTATHIONE** is considered to be the most important **IntraCellular** defense against damage by **Reactive Oxygen Species (ROS)**.

*** BETA CAROTENE** – is a **Carotenoid** that works in Synergy with **Vitamin E.**

A diet **LOW** in Natural Good **FATS**, impairs the absorption of **Beta Carotene** and **Vitamin E** and other **Fat-Soluble Nutrients**.

Fruits and **Vegetables** are our Naturally created sources of **Vitamin C** and **Carotenoids**.

Whole Grains and **High Quality Vegetable Oils** (Coconut, Olive, Flaxseed, etc) are Major sources of **Vitamin E.**

Phenolic compounds such as **FLAVONOIDS** are have Good **Anti-Oxidant** Properties. **Flavonoids** are found Abundantly in several **Fruits** and **Vegetables**.

ALL these Food sources REQUIRE an Oxygen Sufficient Environment in order to be fully utilized by our Bodies.

Chapter 16 ... OxyGen - Healing & Health

*****

During Exercising, **Nasal** Breathing causes a **Reduction** in **FEO2**, which indicates that on **Expiration**, the percentage of **Oxygen** extracted from the **Air** by the **Lungs** is **Increased** and an Increase in **FECO2**- indicating that also on **Expiration**, we have an **Increase** in Expired **Air** that is **Carbon Dioxide**. This is how in combination with physical activities and proper Respiration work to increase the level of Oxygen in Self.

The first place **Blood** (Oxygen rich or deficient) travels to is the **Brain**. The ability to control Self, mind and body, is dependent on **Oxygen**-rich **Blood**.

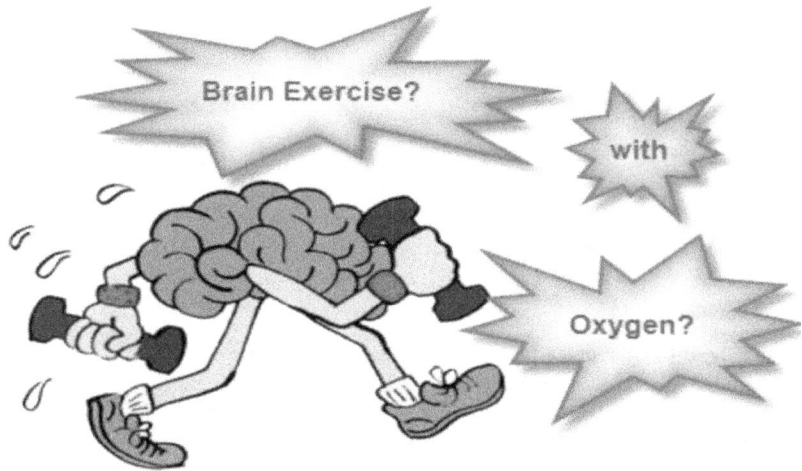

The Brain is the Control-center and therefore all actions within self is based on the Activity of the Brain. This includes Voluntary and Involuntary Body functions, from Heartbeat, to Breathing, to Walking and Thinking.

Oxygen is also proven to be effective in wound healing. This is because we are made of **Cells** and each **Cell** needs it's own Source of **Oxygen** to stay **ALIVE**. When they have sufficient **Oxygen** to function normally – **Heal** at a normal rate.

*****Oxygen** is necessary to increase **Cell Metabolism** and **Energy** production. **Oxygen** is required for **Cell** survival and production of **Molecules**, **Movement** and to **Transport Energy**.

*****Oxygen** is necessary to increase the Rate of Cell Reproduction and Re-Epithelization.

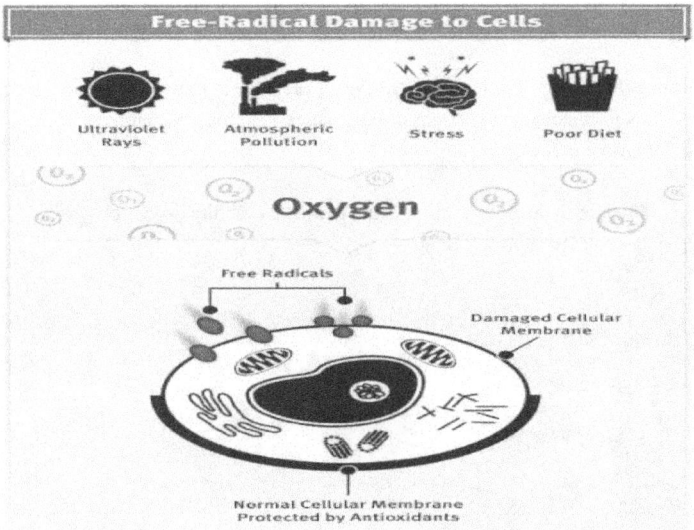

Epithelial Cells line the **Major Cavities** of our **Body**. They come in form the Side of a wound and form a barrier between the wound and environment. This is the foundation for forming **NEW SKIN** !

*****Oxygen** is necessary to create **Collagen** and Increase **Tensile Strength**. **Oxygen** is essential to make and properly Organize **Collagen**, which is the primary component of **Skin**. **Collagen** accounts for **70-80%** (Dry weight) and acts as a Structural scaffold of **Skin**. Organized **Collagen** is bundled into **Fibers** (like strands of a rope), which are inter-woven and can be stretched in multiple directions without tearing.

Collagen is the Main Structural component in the **Extra-Cellular** space in our various **Connective Tissues.** As the main component of **Connective Tissue, Collagen** is the most abundant **Protein** in us, making up **25-30%** of whole-body **Protein** content.

Tensile Strength is a measurement of the **Force** required to break something.

*****Oxygen** is necessary to increase **Anti-Bacterial** activities. **Oxygen** is essential for Respiratory Burst – the production of **Reactive Oxygen Species (ROS)** that's used by **PHAGOCYTES, NEUTROPHILS** and **MACROPHAGES** (good guys) in Disinfectant Activities and the removal of **Necrotic Cellular** debris.

*****Oxygen** is necessary to create **ANGIOGENESIS.** Angiogenesis is the creation of NEW **BLOOD VESSELS.** These New **Blood Vessels** in-turn Promotes NEW **BLOOD CIRCULATION.** These are essential to **Growth** and Survival of **Repair Tissue.**

*****Oxygen** is necessary to Promote **GROWTH Factors** in the signaling of **Skin Formation.** The **ROS** are essential for the signaling processes of **Skin Formation.**

Lactic Acid is the Direct By-Product of being **Oxygen Deficient.** It is mainly produced by the **Muscle Tissues** and **Red Blood Cells. Lactic Acid** is also a '**Back-up**' to ensure that we can continue to produce **ENERGY** in an **ANAEROBIC** State (Without **Oxygen**).

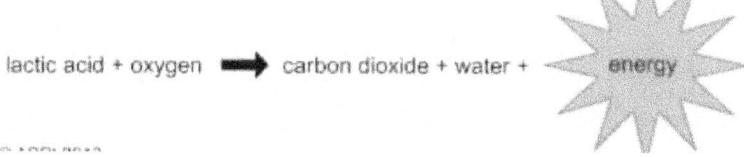

lactic acid + oxygen ➡ carbon dioxide + water + energy

Glucose is our **Energy** Source. It is stored in our **Bodies**, with the highest concentrations in our **Muscles**, in the form of **GLYCOGEN** to be used for **Energy.** During Strenuous Movements,

Exercise or High-Levels of Stress/Anxiety, our **Bodies** uses **Oxygen** to convert the stored **Glycogen** into **ATP**. **ATP** is the **Energy** used to Support our **Muscle** System to KEEP us Moving.

The longer we are under Strenuous Movements our **Bodies** are unable to Keep-Up With and Supply the demands for **Oxygen** and **Energy**.

Our **Glycogen** and **Oxygen** Levels are **Depleted** and our **Cells** change from **Aerobic Respiration** INTO **Anaerobic Respiration (WITHOUT Oxygen)**, in order to **KEEP MOVING.**

LOW Glycogen Levels produce the condition of **GLYCOLYSIS**. Glycolysis is a Process of **12 Chemical Reactions** that produces **Lactic Acid** thru the **GLYCOLITIC Energy** Pathway.
*The Word Equation - **GLUCOGEN** > **GLUCOSE** > **PYRUVIC ACID** > **INSUFFICIENT OXYGEN** > **LACTIC ACID** > ADP+P > ATP > **ENERGY**

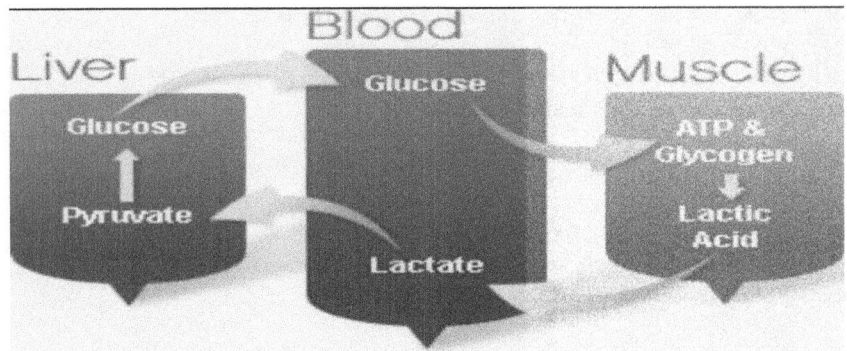

This **Lactic Acid** acts as **Safety Precaution** and **Energy** Source to keep our **Muscles** and **Body** from **Contractile Failure** - when we keep ourselves in a continual state of High Tension, Stress, Movement without **REST** and Proper **Oxygen** Levels.

The **Energy** generated by **Lactic Acid** provides only a quick supply of Short-Bursts of **ATP** to the **Body**. This lasts between **30-60 Seconds** and **3 Minutes** on occasions.

If **Lactic Acid** does not **BURN** when produced-used, it will **Build-Up** around the **Cell** and Clog the **Cell**, depriving it of **Oxygen**.

Lactic Acid also Builds-Up and Clogs **Arteries** and **Veins** – Negatively affecting **Blood Pressure** and **Flow**. This **Build-Up** of **Lactic Acid** is called **LACTIC ACID FERMENTATION**.

Lactic Acid Fermentation is a type of **Anaerobic Respiration** where **SUGARS** and **STARCHES** replace **Oxygen** (The **Breath of LIFE**) for **Fuel**.

The Break-Down and Removal of **Lactic Acid** takes up to **2 Hours** - under **Proper Oxygen** Levels.

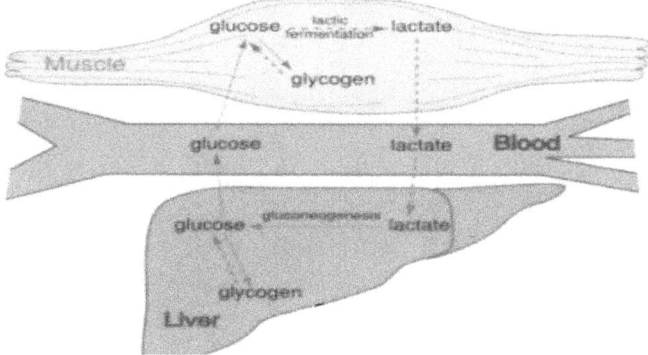

Very High levels of **Lactic Acid** can cause the potential life-threatening Reaction – **Lactic Acidosis**.

The **LIVER** is responsible for filtering **Lactic Acid** out of our **Bodies**. It is the main **Organ** Damaged from **Lactic Acidosis** which are the reaction of us Inhaling incorrectly.

BREATHING TEST

Lie on your back and put one hand on top of your chest and one on top of your stomach. Take a deep breath and see which hand moves.

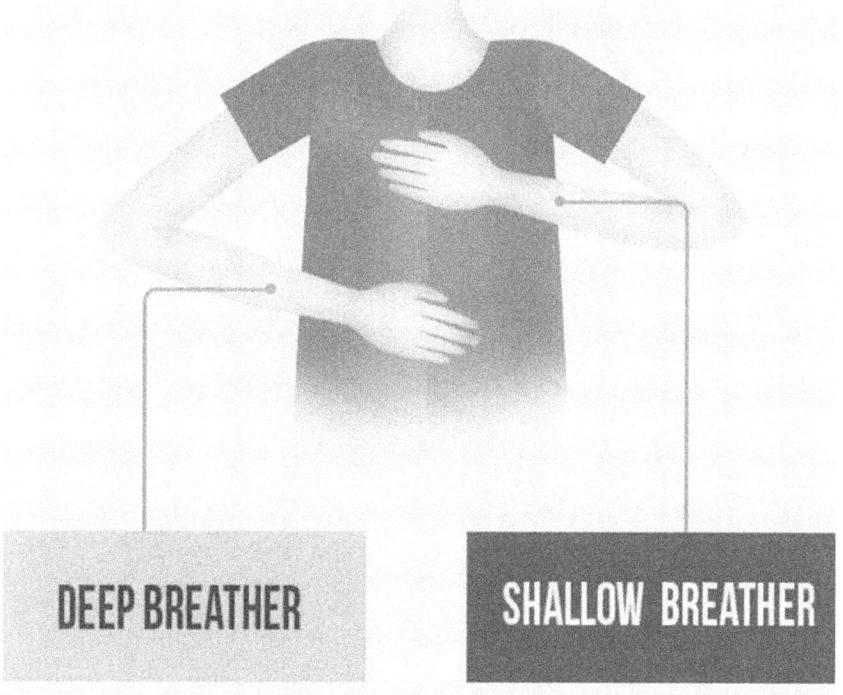

OxyGen ... The Breath Of Life In Atomic Form!

Chapter 17 ... Conscious Breathing

*****

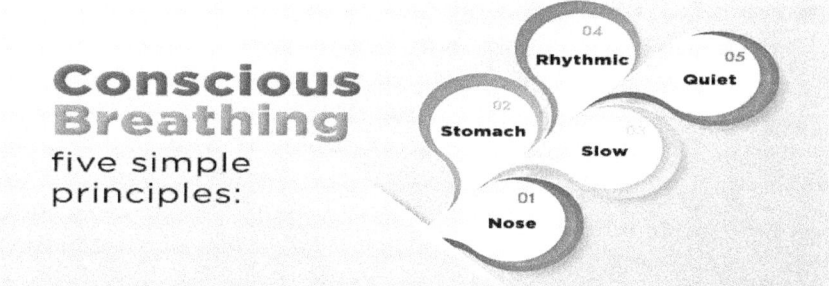

Since we all lose our Natural Breathing Rhythm and Patterns by age 5, becoming a Conscious Breather is critical to regaining and returning to our Natural God Form.

Conscious Breathing is the act of understanding HOW to Properly Inhale, Utilize and Exhale the Breath Of Life that we may BE Living Souls !!

There are 5 easy and natural steps to accomplishing Conscious Breathing :

    1.   *The NOSE*. Knowing and understanding the Respiratory system, parts and functions is the 1st step. The Nose is the ONLY Point of entrance and exit of our Respiratory system. The Mouth is for EMERGENCY RESPIRATION ONLY.

    2.   *The STOMACH*. The Diaphragm is the Organ that inflates the Lungs and the Stomach aides in the proper function of the Diaphragm. Majority of the improper Respiration involves Chest (Swallow) breathing which is detrimental because the Lungs aren't inflated to capacity. The Stomach should move when breathing properly.

3. **_SLOW_**. The average Heartbeat should register between 60 -75 bpm. Our breathing controls our rate and intensity of our heartbeat. Improper breathing (mouth and chest) causes a continuously fast heartbeat that causes Stress and wear on the Heart = premature death.

4. **_The RYTHYM._** Finding and functioning according to our God-Created Natural Breathing RYTHYM is the Key to Health and Wellness. The Breath Of Life (Oxygen) is the Life Force of our physical existence. Breathing according to our God RYTHYM gives us the Ability to BE !!

5. **_QUIET_**. This represents the Awareness and Ability to silence the distractive noises of our environments and be able to Focus on the Quietness of Conscious Breathing !

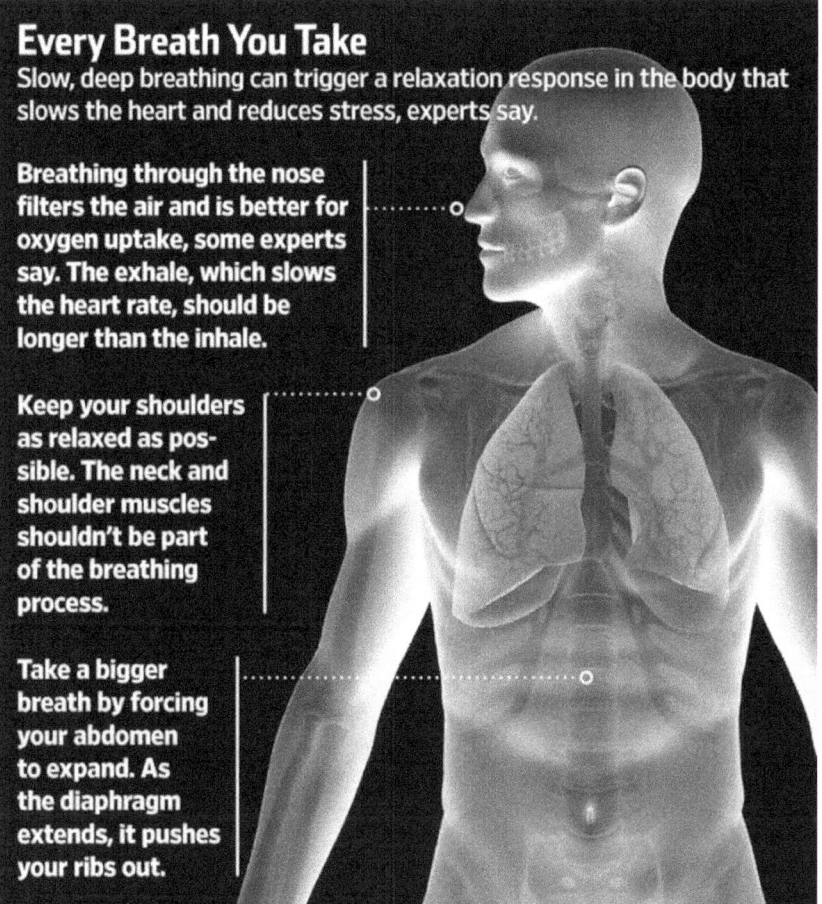

Every Breath You Take

Slow, deep breathing can trigger a relaxation response in the body that slows the heart and reduces stress, experts say.

Breathing through the nose filters the air and is better for oxygen uptake, some experts say. The exhale, which slows the heart rate, should be longer than the inhale.

Keep your shoulders as relaxed as possible. The neck and shoulder muscles shouldn't be part of the breathing process.

Take a bigger breath by forcing your abdomen to expand. As the diaphragm extends, it pushes your ribs out.

OxyGen ... The Breath Of Life In Atomic Form!

HOW DOES ONE BECOME A CONSCIOUS BREATHER ??

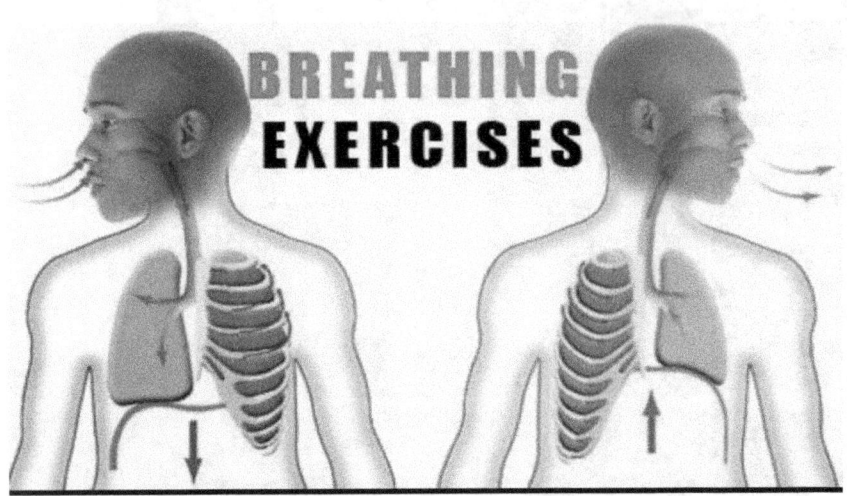

From a health standpoint, **Cardiorespiratory Endurance Activity** is about as close as you can get to an **elixir** for **physical health** and **well-being**. It can help you lose weight, ease stress, boost your immune system, and reduce the risk of certain diseases. Of **ALL** the Organs and/or Systems that comprise our bodies….the **ONLY** one that is used for Life (what it's based on and how we save) is the **Heart** and **Respiratory System**.

    As we have looked at the major organ and systems throughout this book, the **Heart** is the **Life Engine**….we can literally continue to live without any other organ except the Heart.

The **ONLY** organ that we judge our base **Life or Death** on is the **Heart** …. It's Beat and Pressure!

    So, as we look to **Effectively** and **Efficiently Build** our **Supreme Health**, we have to **Start** with the **Life Organ** – The **HEART** and **Cardiorespiratory System**!

OxyGen ... The Breath Of Life In Atomic Form!

Once we have adequately **Strengthened** and **Built** our **Heart** and **Cardiorespiratory** system, we can significantly Increase the capabilities of our Bodies to **Successfully Move** and **Carry** us into **Enjoying Abundant Life**!

Cardiorespiratory Endurance Activity: Exercise that contracts large muscle groups and increases breathing and heart rate.

Aerobic exercise: Exercise that depends on oxygen for energy production.

Merriam-Webster's Dictionary defines *aerobic* as "occurring only in the presence of oxygen." Linked with exercise, *aerobic* refers to any activity that increases oxygen intake and heart rate and keeps them elevated for at least 20 minutes.

When you exercise aerobically, you repeatedly contract large muscle groups, such as your legs and arms, and increase your breathing and your heart rate.

Yoga, Tai Chi, Pilates, Martial Arts and Meditations apply Proper Breathing techniques to Heal, Calm, Exercise, Train and Build our Respiratory system and improved all the Systems and Organs of Self with particular focus placed on Mental Clarity, Health and Wellness.

Each of the above mentioned sciences show the importance of the Breath Of Life and how proper Respiration as a tremendously Life-Giving charge to our Life.

Staying Aware of HOW we are Inhaling and Exhaling is the root of Conscious Breathing. Both the Inhale and Exhale are just as vital and necessary to be performed properly.

The Inhale bring IN Fresh, Pure and Clean Breath Of Life.

The Exhale is when we 'USE' the Breath Of Life and release the Life Energy contained within its Atomic Bonds.

For Every Action there is an Opposite and Equal Re-Action. The Act of improper Respiration causes an Oxygen deficient (Lack of Breath Of Life) environment within Self – that dis-eases, bacteria, viruses and cancers function at.

The Act of proper Respiration creates an Oxygen rich Body (Maximum Breath Of Life), that allows us to successfully Build and Maintain our own Supreme Health and Fitness.

We are created with a Body that can literally last forever. The Breath Of Life in the Atomic form of Oxygen is our LIFE FUEL & ENERGY – ONLY with proper performance!

Posture & Breathing

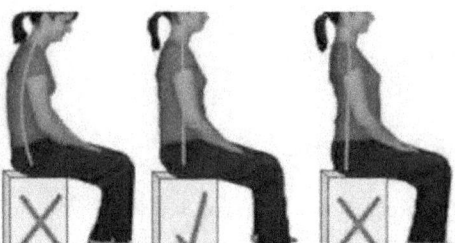

Sitting with straight back
Shoulders relaxed
Diaphragm free, not crushed
Relaxed, comfortable and balanced

Avoid sleeping on your back, this tends to increase breathing rate, lie on the left side (the best position to reduce breathing), right side or stomach.

Posture is just as critical to successful **Respiration** as is proper use of the Diaphragm. When sitting, a majority of people sit in a position that decreases and inhibits the circulation of our **Blood Flow** and **Pressure** which causes deficiency in our **Oxygen** level. **Oxygen** is circulated through the **Blood** stream. The better and stronger Blood pressure and flow are, equates to a higher level of Oxygenation in self.

- Exercise helps move more oxygen to the brain.
- Exercise has been shown to increase levels of BDNF.
- BDNF increases the number of nerve cells in the hippocampas.

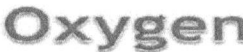
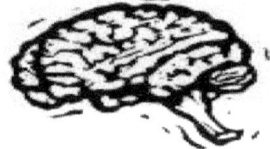

CardioRespiratory Fitness (CRF)

There is absolutely no question that higher levels of physical activity and CRF are associated with reduced risks of chronic diseases and death from all causes. Consequently, it is important to focus on a healthy level of CRF as a lifelong goal that makes life more enjoyable as well as healthy. Those benefits alone merit the inclusion of CRF in any discussion about positive health.

CRF, also called *Cardiovascular* or *Aerobic Fitness*, is a good measure of the heart's ability to pump Oxygen-rich Blood to our Muscles. Although the terms **Cardio** (Heart), **Vascular** (Blood Vessels), **Respiratory** (Lungs and Ventilation), and **Aerobic** (working with Oxygen) differ technically, they all reflect aspects of CRF.

A person with a healthy Heart that can pump great volumes of Blood with each beat has a high level of CRF.

Why Test Cardiorespiratory Fitness?

Results from CRF tests are used to write exercise recommendations and allow the fitness professional or physician to evaluate positive or negative changes in CRF resulting from physical conditioning, aging, illness, or inactivity.

Given the current increase in obesity and inactivity in people of all ages, it makes sense to evaluate CRF throughout life, from early childhood to old age.

This information can indicate where individuals stand on health-criterion tests, and it alerts them to subtle changes in lifestyle that may compromise positive health. The nature of the tests and the level of monitoring should vary across age groups to reflect the information that is needed.

CRF testing depends on the purposes of the test, the type of person to be evaluated, and the work tasks available. Reasons for testing include:

- determining physiological responses at rest and during submaximal or maximal work,

- providing a basis for exercise programming,

- evaluating the effectiveness of one's training program,

- screening for CHD, and

- determining a person's ability to perform a specific work task.

OxyGen ... The Breath Of Life In Atomic Form!

Your Heart Rate Test

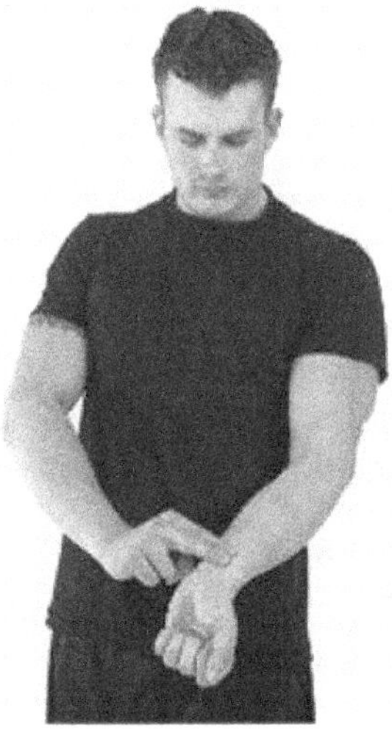

Activity 1: *Measuring Your Heart Rate*

1. Use your fingertips, not your thumb, to find your pulse at the radial artery (at your wrist, below your thumb).

2. Count the beats for 15 seconds.

3. Multiply this number by 4 to get your heart rate in beats per minute (bpm).

Note: Some prefer other methods, such as the following:

a. Count the beats for 10 seconds and multiply by 6 to get the heart rate.

b. Count the beats for 30 seconds and multiply by 2 to get the heart rate.

c. Count the beats for 6 seconds and multiply by 10 to get the heart rate.

Caution: Some prefer feeling the carotid artery in the neck. Your heart's rhythm may be affected if the carotid artery is felt, massaged, or rubbed.

For each of the methods, record your resting heart rate.

<u>15 seconds × 4 =</u> _____

<u>10 seconds × 6 =</u> _____

<u>30 seconds × 2 =</u> _____

<u> 6 seconds × 10 =</u> _____

OxyGen ... The Breath Of Life In Atomic Form!

Determining Your Target Heart Rate Range - Maximum Heart Rate (HRmax) Method

The heat rate provides a convenient way to monitor exercise intensity. Cardiorespiratory fitness will not increase unless the heart rate during exercise rises to at least a predetermined minimum level. This level is known as the target heart rate range and is about 60% to 80% of the maximum heart rate (maximum heart rate is the highest number of times your heart can beat in 1 minute). When you exercise, you should strive to keep your heart rate inside this range.

Use your findings from the previous Heart Rate test for determining your heart rate for 1 minute. Complete the chart below to derive your target heart rate range (low end and high end).

Most people have misinterpreted the target heart rate range, believing that exercise has to be very tense or it is useless. This is not true, but the belief discourages many from participating in, and benefiting from, exercise.

Example of with resting heart rate of 70 at 60% to 80% training range:

Low end	High end
HRmax = 208 − (0.7 × age)	HRmax = 208 − (0.7 × age)
HRmax = 208 − (0.7 × 25) = 190.5	HRmax = 208 − (0.7 × 25) = 190.5
HRR = HRmax − HRrest	HRR = HRmax − HRrest
HRR = 190.5 − 70 = 120.5	HRR = 190.5 − 70 = 120.5
Low-end target range % = HRR × intensity % + HRrest	High-end target range % = HRR × intensity % + HRrest
60% intensity = 120.5 × 0.60 + 70 = 142 bpm	80% intensity = 120.5 × 0.80 + 70 = 166 bpm

Age = _____

Resting heart rate (HRrest) = _____

Low-end intensity level = _____

High-end intensity level = _____

Low end	High end
HRmax =	HRmax =
HRR =	HRR =
Low-end target range pulse per minute =	Low-end target range pulse per minute =

Key to abbreviations:

HRmax = Maximum heart rate

HRR = Heart rate reserve

HRrest = Resting heart rate

bpm = beats per minute

OxyGen ... The Breath Of Life In Atomic Form!

Benefits of Cardiorespiratory Endurance Exercise

*****

Regular endurance exercise can benefit the body in many healthy ways. Following are the short- and long-term benefits achieved by exercising regularly, using the cardiorespiratory system. **Short-Term Benefits**

Many people start a physical activity program because of its long-term benefits; however, it is the short-term benefits that keep them motivated to continue the habit.

Relaxes and Revitalizes

Physical activity reduces mental and muscular tension and increases concentration and energy levels. Regular aerobic exercise releases **endorphins**.

Endorphins: Proteins produced in your brain that serve as your body's natural pain-killer. Endorphins also reduce stress, depression, and anxiety.

Offers a Break from Daily Routine and Stress. Planned or unplanned physical activity can be enjoyable and provide a release from dayto-day stress and boredom.

Helps You Feel Good About Yourself. Physical activity can improve your self-esteem and self-confidence, and enhance your general sense of well-being.

Long-Term Benefits

Decreases Risk of Heart Disease. The **leading health threat today is cardiovascular disease, which includes heart attack, stroke, hypertension, coronary artery disease** (the buildup of fatty deposits on the inside of arteries), and congestive heart failure. Coronary artery disease (also called heart disease) and stroke are major causes of disability.

Prevents plaque buildup in arteries. Atherosclerosis is another key factor in cardiovascular disease. Fatty deposits called plaques build up as particles of low-density lipoprotein (LDL, or "bad" cholesterol) pass out of the bloodstream and lodge in weakened portions of artery walls, including the arteries supplying the heart and the brain. Over time, these plaques can narrow the vessels enough to deprive these organs of oxygen-rich blood. When this happens in the heart, it can lead to a heart attack. Blocked arteries in the brain can result in a stroke.

Moderate to vigorous aerobic exercise increases healthy high-density lipoprotein (HDL) cholesterol in our blood. HDL transports fats back to your liver for metabolism, preventing their accumulation along artery walls. Exercise also reduces the blood levels of unhealthy LDL cholesterol and triglycerides.

Protects arteries. **Exercise can help keep arteries resilient.** Regular expansion and contraction of arteries during exercise keeps the vessels "in shape."

Makes clots less likely. **Exercise helps keep the inner lining of the arteries healthy and thereby less prone to injuries that set the stage for plaque formation.** It also inhibits clot formation by making platelets less "sticky" and promotes the release of enzymes that break down clots. Higher activity levels lower inflammation in the arteries.

Promotes new coronary arteries. **Aerobic exercise can lead to an increase in the size and number of coronary arteries feeding the heart.** If an arterial blockage occurs, there is less risk of heart muscle damage because there are alternative channels to keep the blood supply flowing. Women's bone density is typically greatest in their mid-20s to mid-30s, but then declines slowly until menopause, which is a time of rapid bone loss. Physical activity in younger years will help women maintain good bone mass at menopause. **Even physical activity begun later in life or during menopause will help slow the loss of bone.**

Decreases Risk of Cancer. **Exercise increases circulation and respiration, accelerates the movement of food through the bowels, improves energy metabolism and immune function, and affects hormone levels.** All of these may help protect against most types of cancer.

Lowers Blood Pressure. **Exercise helps protect you from cardiovascular disease in numerous ways.** The less active you are, the more likely you are to develop hypertension. Chronic hypertension doubles or triples the risk for developing congestive heart failure and can lead to heart disease, brain hemorrhage, aortic aneurysms, kidney disease and failure, and damage to other organs.

Increases Stamina. Exercise may cause fatigue immediately after the activity. Over the long term, though, it will increase stamina and reduce fatigue.

Lowers Body Fat. Exercise can counter creeping weight gain. Approximately 70% of the energy burned every day is taken up by bodily functions; the remaining 30% depends on our level of activity, so exercise choices certainly make a difference.

For people who are already overweight, exercise is an integral part of any weight-loss program. The most effective way to lose weight is to increase your level of activity and to reduce the calories you consume.

Cutting back on calories leads to faster weight loss than from exercising. Because you need to burn 3500 calories to lose a single pound, it may take a few weeks of regular, moderate exercise to successfully do so. However, consuming 500 less calories a day will result in the loss of a pound a week.

If you only cut back on calories, however, you are more likely to regain the weight lost. That is because your body reacts to weight loss as if it were starving and, in response, slows its metabolism. When your metabolism slows, you burn less calories. Increasing your physical activity will counteract the metabolic slowdown caused by reducing calories.

Exercise raises your energy expenditure while you are exercising and also while you are resting when the workout is done. Pounds lost by increasing your activity level consist almost entirely of fat.

Improves Muscular Health. Aerobic exercise stimulates the growth of blood vessels and capillaries in the muscles, providing for more efficient oxygen delivery to the muscles and helping to remove irritating metabolic waste products such as lactic acid. This can reduce pain in those who have fibromyalgia and chronic low-back pain.

Reduces the Number of Sick Days. Many studies report that people who exercise regularly are less susceptible to minor viral illnesses, such as colds or flu, because of an improved immune system.

Decreases the Chance of Premature Death. In 1986, results from the Harvard Alumni Health Study published in the *New England Journal of Medicine* for the first time linked exercise with increased life spans. Since then, additional research has supported this finding.

Decreases Cholesterol and Triglyceride Levels. High blood cholesterol and triglyceride levels increase the risk of heart disease. Regular exercise raises the level of good cholesterol (HDL), which may help to clear blood vessels and to lower the level of bad cholesterol (LDL). HDLs and LDLs are discussed further in the text.

Decreases the Risk of Diabetes. Untreated or poorly treated diabetes can lead to blindness, kidney disease, and the loss of limbs. It is also a major factor in heart disease and stroke.

All Cells need **sugar** as a source of **energy**. Insulin, a **hormone** produced by the **Pancreas, helps cells extract sugar from the blood**. When you have **diabetes**, your body is **unable to make or use insulin efficiently**, so you have **excess sugar** (Glucose) in your blood. About **5% to 10%** of people with diabetes **cannot make insulin at all**; this condition is called **Type 1 diabetes**. Those who have **Type 1 diabetes** must take daily insulin shots.

<u>**Type 2 diabetes**</u> accounts for **90% to 95%** of cases of diabetes. In **Type 2 diabetes, the pancreas can pump out more insulin for a time, but eventually it cannot keep up with the greater demand, and blood glucose levels rise.** Type 2 diabetes often can be controlled by diet and exercise, although medications or insulin may eventually be needed.

Type-2 diabetes: A disease that involves the inability to produce an adequate amount of insulin.

Obesity: Excessive amounts of body fat.

Exercise lowers modest amounts of blood glucose and boosts the body's sensitivity to insulin. This can help control existing diabetes and, most important, stave off the onset of type 2 diabetes.

Decreases the Risk of Osteoporosis. **Weight-bearing exercise is necessary to stimulate the growth of new bone tissue.** When demands are put on a bone, it responds by becoming stronger and denser.

Any activity that works against gravity can potentially build Bone. Examples of such activities include running, walking, weight lifting, and stair climbing. However, activities such as swimming or biking, which are not weight-bearing, do not build bone. Higher-impact activities or resistance exercises (e.g., strength training) have a greater effect on bone than lower-impact exercises (e.g., walking) do. Only the bone that actually bears the load of the exercise will benefit, however. For example, walking or running protects bones in the lower extremities. A well-rounded strength training plan can help all of your bones.

Decreases Arthritis Symptoms. **Overuse of certain joints can set the stage for arthritis, but regular moderate activity does not raise the risk for this disease developing in normal joints.** Instead, moderate exercise—whether aerobic or resistance—actually helps to reduce swelling in joints and relieve pain. When joints are not used, the cartilage thins and softens, making the joint more vulnerable to arthritis. Exercise can also control weight. Overweight and **obesity** put people at a much higher risk for developing arthritis.

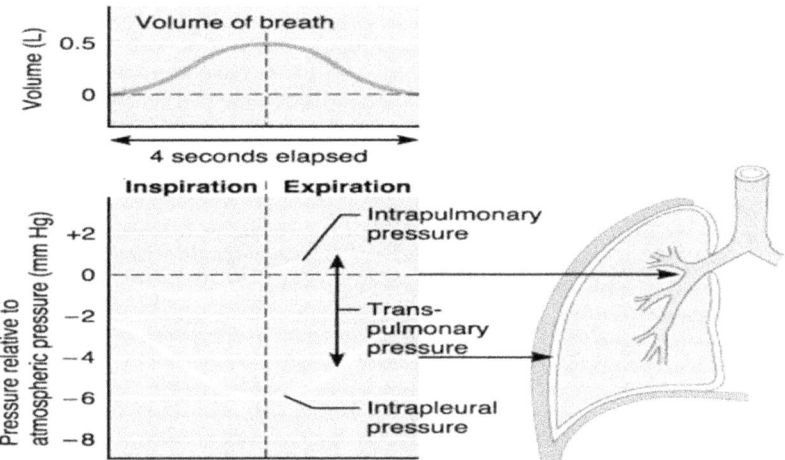

OxyGen ... The Breath Of Life In Atomic Form!

Supreme Health Cardiorespiratory Health Assessments

*****

Activity 1: Supreme Health - Fitness Walking Test™

This activity assesses **cardiorespiratory** (aerobic) fitness. To perform the test, you need a watch with a second hand to record your time, and you need to wear good walking shoes and loose clothes. You should have your physician's consent before undertaking this exercise test.

Instructions:

1. Find a measured track or measure 1 mile using your car's odometer on a level, uninterrupted road.

2. Warm-up by walking slowly for 5 minutes.

3. 1 mile as fast as you can, maintaining a steady pace. Note the time that you began walking.

4. When you complete the mile walk, record your time to the nearest second and keep walking at a slower pace. Count your pulse for 15 seconds and multiply by 4, then record this number. This gives your heart rate per minute after your test walk.

*Heart rate at the end of 1-mile walk: _____ beats per minute.

*Time to walk the mile: _____ minutes.

5. Remember to stretch once you have cooled down.

6. To find your cardiorespiratory fitness level, refer to the appropriate Supreme Health Fitness Walking Test charts based on your age and sex. These show established fitness norms from the American Heart Association.

Using your fitness level chart, find your time in minutes and your heart rate per minute. Follow these lines until they meet, and mark this point on your chart. This tells you how fit you are compared to other individuals of your sex and age category.

These charts are based on weights of 170 lb for men and 125 lb for women. If you weigh substantially less, your cardiovascular fitness will be slightly underestimated. Conversely, if you weigh substantially more, your cardiovascular fitness will be slightly overestimated.

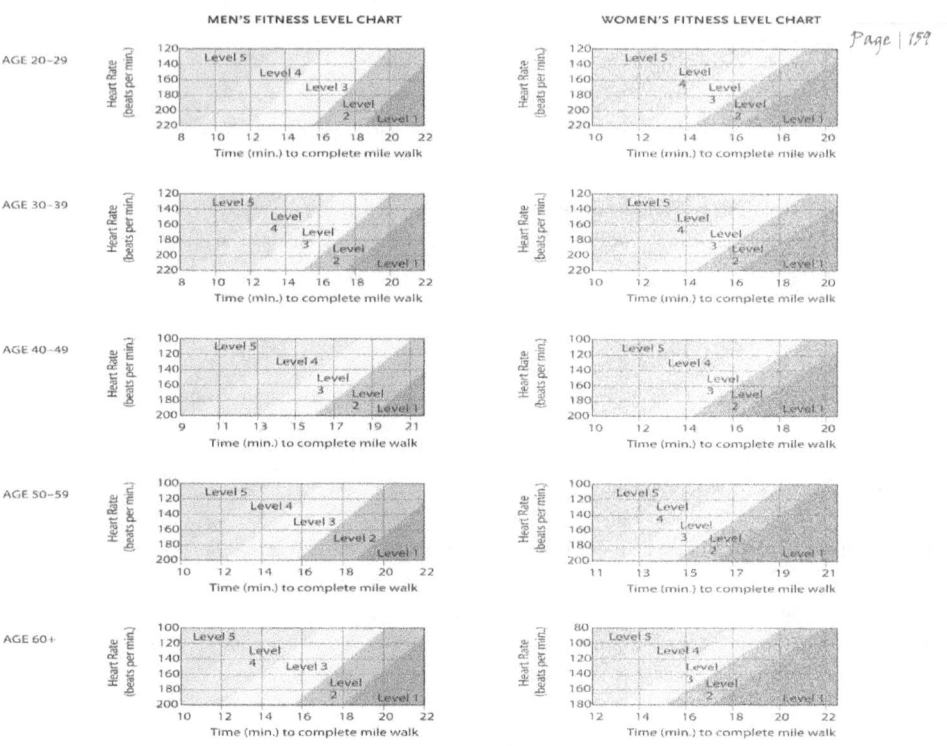

How fit you are compared to others of the same age and gender:

Level 5 = high

Level 4 = above average

Level 3 = average

Level 2 = below average

Level 1 = low

OxyGen ... The Breath Of Life In Atomic Form!

****

Activity 2: *Supreme Health's - 1.5-Mile Run/Walk Test*

The **1.5-mile run/walk** test is recommended for those who are motivated, experienced in running, and in good condition before taking the test. Do not take the test unless you can already jog nonstop for 15 minutes. It is not recommended for the following people:

- Those failing the PAR-Q questionnaire

- Severely Sedentary people older than 30 years of age

- Severely deconditioned people

- Those with joint problems

Sedentary individuals (especially those older than 30 years of age) should participate in a walking/running program for 1 to 2 months before taking the test. For those in hot or cold environments, do not take this test unless you have been exercising in these conditions.

Preparation

You will need the following:

- Stopwatch, watch, or clock with a second hand

- Oval running track

- Appropriate running shoes and clothing

Warm up for 5 to 10 minutes before the test.

Procedure

1. Complete a 1.5-mile distance in the shortest possible time. If outdoors, the test should be conducted in favorable weather conditions. Physically fit individuals can cover the distance either by running or jogging. Less fit individuals can run and jog, but may need to walk some of the time.

2. Attempt to keep a steady pace throughout the test.

3. When completed, record the time (minutes and seconds) to complete the 1.5-mile distance.

*Time to finish the 1.5-mile distance: _____

4. See Table to find your fitness rating.

Fitness rating: _____

Fitness category	Age (years)					
	13–19	20–29	30–39	40–49	50–59	60+
Men						
Very poor	>15:30	>16:00	>16:30	>17:30	>19:00	>20:00
Poor	12:11–15:30	14:01–16:00	14:46–16:30	15:36–17:30	17:01–19:00	19:01–20:00
Average	10:49–12:10	12:01–14:00	12:31–14:45	13:01–15:35	14:31–17:00	16:16–19:00
Good	9:41–10:48	10:46–12:00	11:01–12:30	11:31–13:00	12:31–14:30	14:00–16:15
Excellent	8:37–9:40	9:45–10:45	10:00–11:00	10:30–11:30	11:00–12:30	11:15–13:59
Superior	<8:37	<9:45	<10:00	<10:30	<11:00	<11:15
Women						
Very poor	>18:30	>19:00	>19:30	>20:00	>20:30	>21:00
Poor	16:55–18:30	18:31–19:00	19:01–19:30	19:31–20:00	20:01–20:30	20:31–21:31
Average	14:31–16:54	15:55–18:30	16:31–19:00	17:31–19:30	19:01–20:00	19:31–20:30
Good	12:30–14:30	13:31–15:54	14:31–16:30	15:56–17:30	16:31–19:00	17:31–19:30
Excellent	11:50–12:29	12:30–13:30	13:00–14:30	13:45–15:55	14:30–16:30	16:30–18:00
Superior	<11:50	<12:30	<13:00	<13:45	<14:30	<16:30

Activity 3: Supreme Health & Fitness Step Test

Complete the PAR-Q questionnaire. **Do not take the test if you suffer joint problems in your ankles, knees, or hips, or if you are extremely obese.**

Preparation

You will need the following:

- 12-inch-high sturdy bench
- Metronome
- Stopwatch, watch, or clock with a second hand

Warm up for 5 minutes before taking the test. Practice before, but you should be well rested with no prior exercise of any kind for several hours before the test.

Procedure

1. Set the metronome at 96 beats per minute (four clicks of the metronome equals one step-cycle: up—1, 2; down—3, 4).

2. Step up and down on the 12-inch bench for 3 minutes.

3. After the 3 minutes of stepping, sit down and within 5 seconds count your radial pulse for 1 full minute.

4. See Table for your fitness rating.

Age (years) Gender	18–25		26–35		36–45	
	Male	Female	Male	Female	Male	Female
Excellent	50–76	52–81	51–76	58–80	49–76	51–84
Good	79–84	85–93	79–85	85–92	80–88	89–96
Above average	88–93	96–102	88–94	95–101	92–98	100–104
Average	95–100	104–110	96–102	104–110	100–105	107–112
Below average	102–107	113–120	104–110	113–119	108–113	115–120
Poor	111–119	122–131	114–121	122–129	116–124	124–132
Very poor	124–157	135–169	126–161	134–171	130–163	137–169

Age (years) Gender	46–55		56–65		Over 65	
	Male	Female	Male	Female	Male	Female
Excellent	56–82	63–91	60–77	60–92	59–81	70–92
Good	87–93	95–101	86–94	97–103	87–92	96–101
Above average	95–101	104–110	97–100	106–111	94–102	104–111
Average	103–111	113–118	103–109	113–118	104–110	116–121
Below average	113–119	120–124	111–117	119–127	114–118	123–126
Poor	121–126	121–132	119–128	129–135	121–126	128–133
Very poor	131–159	137–171	131–154	141–174	130–151	135–155

Activity 4: Cardiorespiratory Training Log

Track your Energy by recording the date, activity, intensity & duration for each workout.

Date	Activity	Intensity (heart rate)	Duration (time)	Comments (e.g., rating of perceived exertion, pain, observations)
Sept. 15	Walk/jog	60% of HRR	30 min.	Great being outdoors

References & Resources:

1. American College of Sports Medicine (ACSM). 2006. *ACSM's guidelines for exercise testing and prescription.* 7th ed. Philadelphia: Lippincott Williams & Wilkins.

2. American College of Sports Medicine (ACSM). 2010. *ACSM's guidelines for exercise testing and prescription.* 8th ed. Philadelphia: Lippincott Williams & Wilkins.

3. American College of Sports Medicine (ACSM). 2010. *ACSM's resource manual for guidelines for exercise testing and prescription.* 6th ed. Baltimore: Lippincott Williams & Wilkins.

4. Åstrand, I. 1960. Aerobic work capacity in men and women with special reference to age. *Acta Physiologica Scandinavica* 49(Suppl. 169): 1-92.

5. Åstrand, P.-O. 1979. *Work tests with the bicycle ergometer.* Varberg, Sweden: Monark-Crescent AB.

6. Åstrand, P.-O. 1984. Principles of ergometry and their implications in sport practice. *International Journal of Sports Medicine* 5:102-105.

7. Åstrand, P.-O., and I. Rhyming. 1954. A nomogram for calculation of aerobic capacity (physical fitness) from pulse rate during submaximal work. *Journal of Applied Physiology* 7:218-221.

8. Åstrand, P.-O., and B. Saltin. 1961. Maximal oxygen uptake and heart rate in various types of muscular activity. *Journal of Applied Physiology* 16:977-981.

9. Bailey, D.A., R.J. Shephard, and R.L. Mirwald. 1976. Validation of a self-administered home test of cardiorespiratory fitness. *Canadian Journal of Applied Sports Sciences* 1:67-78.

10. Balke, B. 1963. A simple field test for assessment of physical fitness. In *Civil Aeromedical Research Institute report,* 63-66. Oklahoma City: Civil Aeromedical Research Institute.

11. Balke, B. 1970. *Advanced exercise procedures for evaluation of the cardiovascular system* (Monograph). Milton, WI: Burdick.

12. Baum, W.A. 1961. *Sphygmomanometers, principles and precepts.* New York: Baum.

13. Blair, S.N., H.W. Kohl III, R.S. Paffenbarger Jr., D.G. Clark, K.H. Cooper, and L.W. Gibbons. 1989. Physical fitness and all-cause mortality. *Journal of the American Medical Association* 262:2395-2401.

14. Borg, G. 1998. *Borg's perceived exertion and pain scales.* Champaign, IL: Human Kinetics.

15. Bransford, D.R., and E.T. Howley. 1977. The oxygen cost of running in trained and untrained men and women. *Medicine and Science in Sports* 9:41-44.

16. Bruce, R.A. 1972. Multistage treadmill test of submaximal and maximal exercise. In *Exercise testing and training of apparently healthy individuals: A handbook for physicians,* ed. American Heart Association, 32-34. New York: American Heart Association.

17. Chun, D.M., C.B. Corbin, and R.P. Pangrazi. 2000. Validation of criterion-referenced standards for the mile run and progressive aerobic cardiovascular endurance tests. *Research Quarterly for Exercise and Sport* 71:125-134.

18. Cooper, K.H. 1977. *The aerobics way.* New York: Bantam Books.

19. Cooper Institute for Aerobics Research. 1999. *Fitnessgram test administration manual.* Champaign, IL: Human Kinetics.

20. Daniels, J.T. 1985. A physiologist's view of running economy. *Medicine and Science in Sports and Exercise* 17:332-338.

21. Daniels, J., N. Oldridge, F. Nagle, and B. White. 1978. Differences and changes in VO_2 among young runners 10-18 years of age. *Medicine and Science in Sports* 10:200-203.

22. Ellestad, M. 1994. *Stress testing: Principles and practice.* Philadelphia: Davis.

23. Franks, B.D. 1979. Methodology of the exercise ECG test. In *Exercise electrocardiography: Practical approach,* ed. E.K. Chung, 46-61. Baltimore: Williams & Wilkins.

24. Frohlich, E.D., C. Grim, D.R. Labarthe, M.H. Maxwell, D. Perloff, and W.H. Weidman. 1988. Recommendations for human blood-pressure determination by sphygmoma-nometers. *Circulation* 77:501A-514A.

25. George, J.D., W.J. Stone, and L.N. Burkett. 1997. Non-exercise VO_2max estimation for physically active college students. *Medicine and Science in Sports and Exercise* 29:415-423.

26. Golding, L.A. 2000. *YMCA fitness testing and assessment manual.* 4th ed. Champaign, IL: Human Kinetics.

27. Hagberg, J.M., J.P. Mullin, M.D. Giese, and E. Spitznagel. 1981. Effect of pedaling rate on submaximal exercise responses of competitive cyclists. *Journal of Applied Physiology* 51:447-451.

28. Heil, D.P., P.S. Freedson, L.E. Ahlquist, J. Price, and J.M. Rippe. 1995. Non-exercise regression models to estimate peak oxygen consumption. *Medicine and Science in Sports and Exercise* 27:599-606.

OxyGen ... The Breath Of Life In Atomic Form!

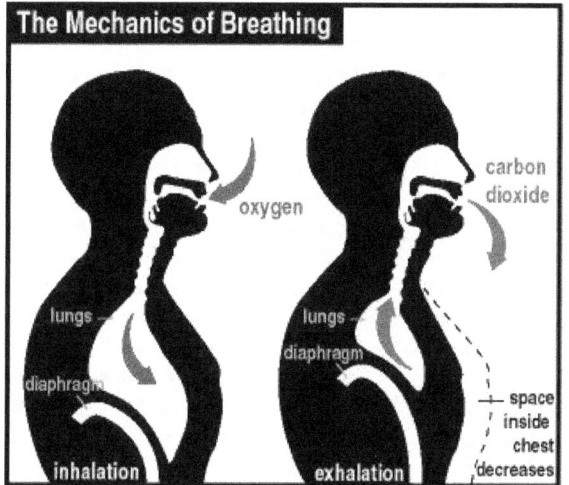

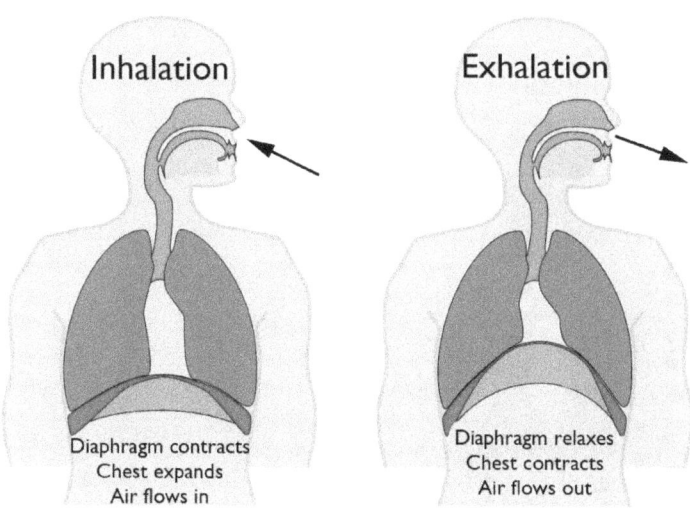

OxyGen ... The Breath Of Life In Atomic Form!

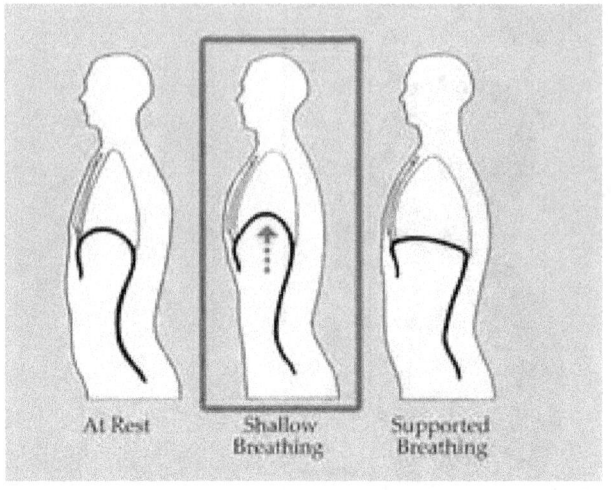

At Rest   Shallow Breathing   Supported Breathing

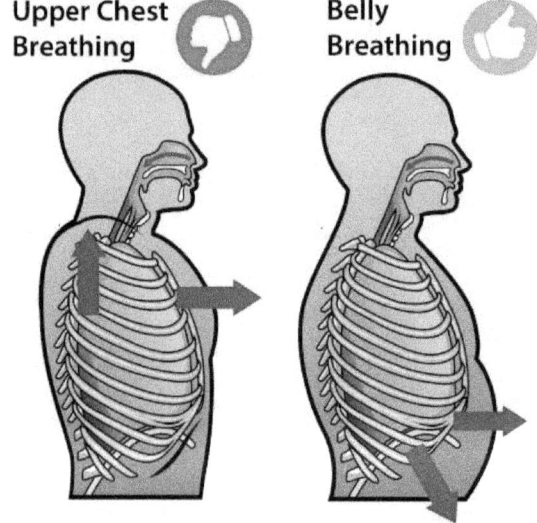

Upper Chest Breathing 👎   **Belly Breathing** 👍

OxyGen ... The Breath Of Life In Atomic Form!

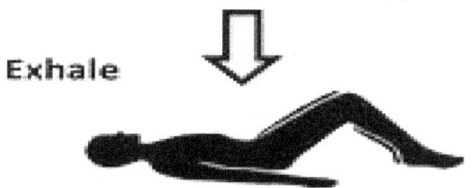

Exhale

Navel draws in toward the spine

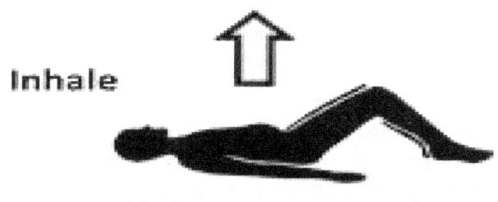

Inhale

Abdomen expands

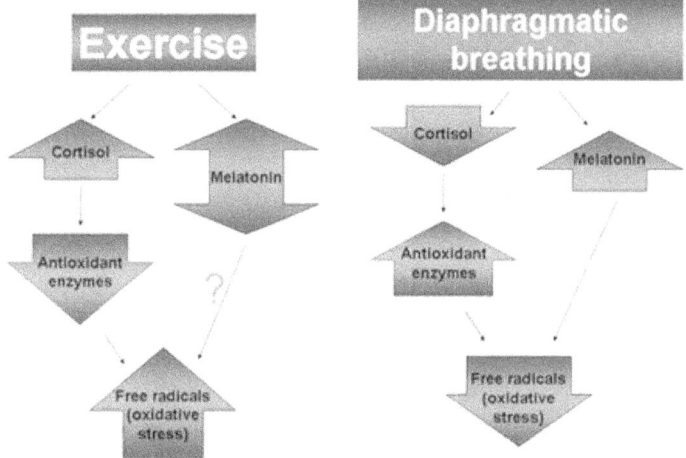

OxyGen... The Breath Of Life In Atomic Form!

BREATHING TEST

Lie on your back and put one hand on top of your chest and one on top of your stomach. Take a deep breath and see which hand moves.

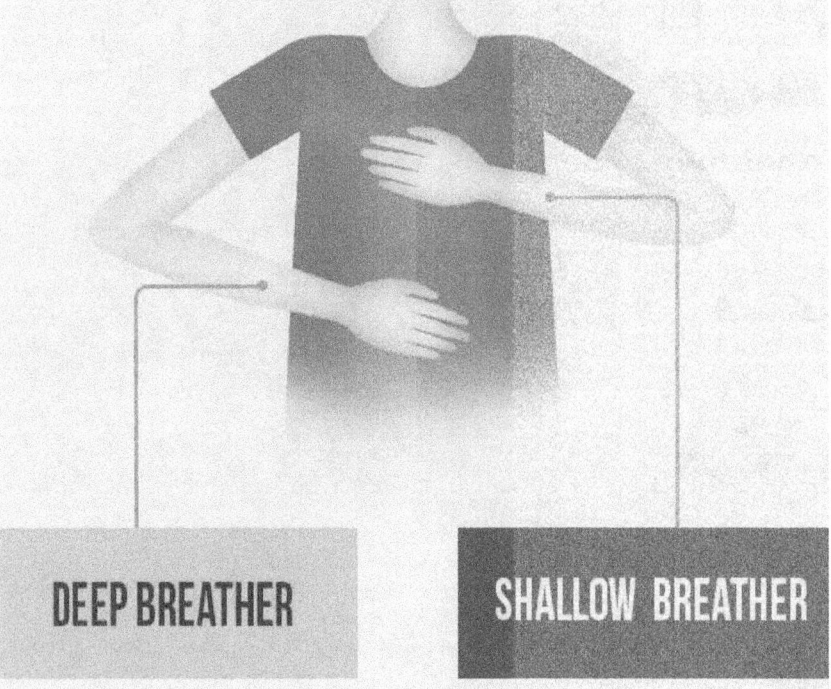

DEEP BREATHER   SHALLOW BREATHER

Benefits of Deeper breathing...
physical

- Increased purification of blood
- Decrease in Toxins
- Increase Digestion
- Decrease Waste
- Improved Nervous System
- Improves functioning the glands, producing chemical requirements of the body
- Improves Lungs capacity & resistance
- Reduces Heart load & makes Heart live longer
- Controls Weight of the body
- Regulate Heat & cooling System of the body
- Improves Health & reduces weakness
- Oxygen to brain & mind relaxes

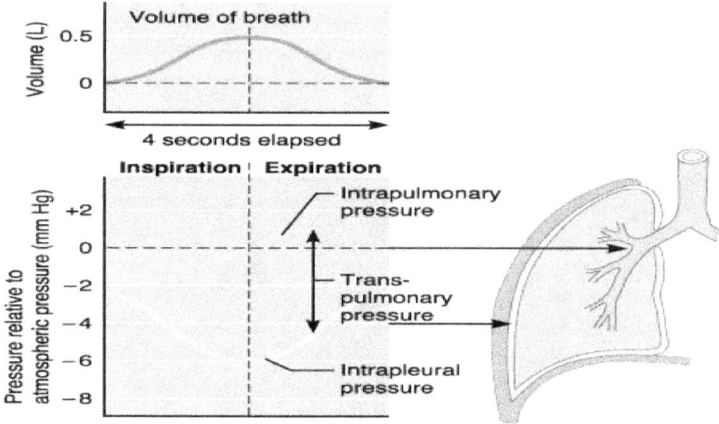

OxyGen ... The Breath Of Life In Atomic Form!

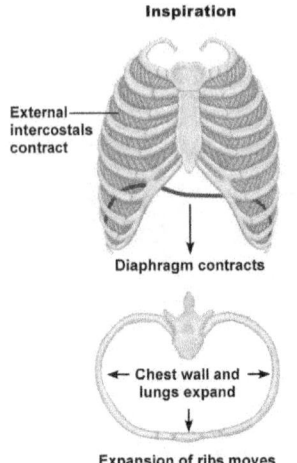
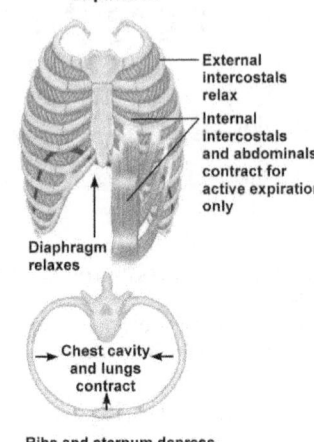
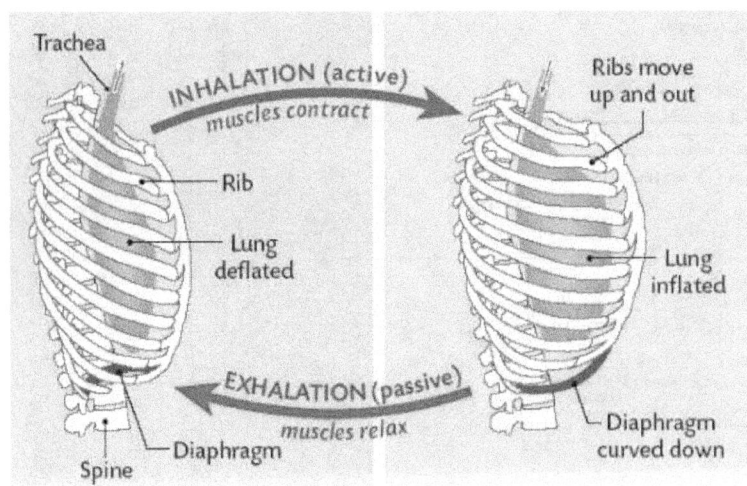

OxyGen ... The Breath Of Life In Atomic Form!

More Publications by Supreme Health and Fitness:

LIFE Energy: The Sun, Glucose & WHY Humans Are Herbivores!
Authored by Sean Ali

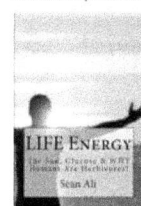

List Price: **$30.00**

6" x 9" (15.24 x 22.86 cm)
Full Color on White paper
156 pages

ISBN-13: **978-1544622842** (CreateSpace-Assigned)
ISBN-10: **1544622848**
BISAC: Medical / Diet Therapy

Peace and Blessings of Health!

*Do YOU have a health issue that YOU would like to over-come?
*Do YOU want to improve the Quality of YOUR Life?
*Do YOU want to experience ABUNDANT LIFE?

*** OPEN THIS BOOK - NOW!!! ***

This small book is written with the purpose of re-examining the role of Nutrition in health care and everyday Life ... LIFE IS ENERGY.... Nutrition is a descriptive term to describe how we replenish our Life Energy.
Understanding Nutrition is the equivalent of understanding Energy
Knowledge of Nutrition enables us to make precise Energy adjustments through Nutrients to provide the proper Energy needed for all our body functions/tasks – from achieving Homeostasis, facilitating our Growth, Development and Self-Healing.
We come from the Earth and all our Solutions are manifested from the Earth..... All we have to do is return back to the Earth and extract what we need
Food is our naturally occurring vehicle, perfectly designed for administering the Life Energy in the form of Nutrition.
Our Food choices and the Energy released from it, presents as either the root cause of our dis-ease or the base for our Solution.
From our Cells to our Immune system, we are Created to Heal and Regenerate Self with the aide of proper Nutrition/Energy.
Our Food is our Medicine ONLY with proper application..... There is no in-between, which means that we are either eating to die – OR – Eating To LIVE !!!
Energy is the Key to LIFE and we Know that the Sun is the Source of all Energy, so if we focus on how to obtain as much Sun in the form of food as possible = the key to Nutritional Health and Therapy
Let us explore and examine Life Energy and how to obtain the best Quality and Value so that we may successfully manifest the Best out of Life and Enjoy a long, active and fruitful Life-span!

Achieving and Maintaining Supreme Health and Fitness by increasing the level of Knowledge and Science of Life!

Peace

OxyGen ... The Breath Of Life In Atomic Form!

Project Summary
Understanding Carbohydrates: LIFE Energy, Fiber, Sugar and Starch!
Authored by Sean Ali

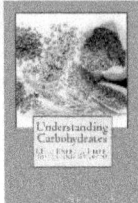

List Price: **$30.00**

6" x 9" (15.24 x 22.86 cm)
Full Color on White paper
150 pages

ISBN-13: **978-1543023763** (CreateSpace-Assigned)
ISBN-10: **1543023762**
BISAC: **Health & Fitness / Healthy Living**

Peace and Blessings of Health!

*Do YOU have health issues that YOU want to over-come?
*Do YOU want to improve the Quality of YOUR Life?
*Do YOU want to experience ABUNDANT LIFE?

*** THEN THIS BOOK IS FOR YOU!! ***

There is a disproportionate amount of fad diets and food-like TOXIC items that are available and which we are bombarded with that promote a detrimentally 'low' or 'no' Carb meal plan that goes TOTALLY against ALL Nutritional science and evidence of the function of Carbohydrates.
There is little to no serious governmental regulation of these types of claims or food-like items and most are cases of clever advertisement vs actual claims of quality and value.
This small book has been produced to provide understanding of the Nutritional and Life value of Carbohydrates - from a Scientific analogy, while simultaneously shedding light on these false claims and food-like products so that YOU can make the Best Life choices for YOUR successful Growth & Development!
Let us explore and learn about our Primary Energy source and become able to make the best Nutritional choices.
OPEN THIS BOOK - and Begin the steps to Successfully Build and Maintain Your own Supreme Health and Fitness!

Peace !
Sean Ali

CreateSpace eStore: https://www.createspace.com/6922679

OxyGen ... The Breath Of Life In Atomic Form!

Project Summary
Enjoying Abundant LIFE!: Scientific Concepts to Successfully Build YOUR Supreme Health!
Authored by Sean Ali

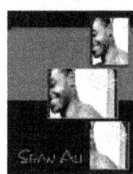

List Price: **$35.00**

8" x 10" (20.32 x 25.4 cm)
Full Color on White paper
170 pages

ISBN-13: 978-1546732075 (CreateSpace-Assigned)
ISBN-10: 1546732071
BISAC: Medical / Healing

Peace and Blessings of Health!

"Do YOU have a health issue that YOU would like to over come?
"Do YOU want to improve the Quality of YOUR Life?
"Do YOU want to experience ABUNDANT LIFE?

*** OPEN THIS BOOK - NOW!!! ***

This small book is written with the purpose of re-examining the role of Nutrition in health care and everyday Life ... LIFE IS ENERGY. ...Nutrition is a descriptive term to describe how we replenish our Life Energy.
Understanding Nutrition is the equivalent of understanding Energy.
Knowledge of Nutrition enables us to make precise Energy adjustments through Nutrients to provide the proper Energy needed for all our body functions/tasks - from achieving Homeostasis, facilitating our Growth, Development and Self Healing.
We come from the Earth and all our Solutions are manifested from the Earth ... All we have to do is return back to the Earth and extract what we need.
Food is our naturally occurring vehicle, perfectly designed for administering the Life Energy in the form of Nutrition.
Our Food choices and the Energy released from it, presents as either the root cause of our dis-ease or the base for our Solution.
From our Cells to our Immune system, we are Created to Heal and Regenerate Self with the aide of proper Nutrition/Energy.
Our Food is our Medicine ONLY with proper application... . There is no in-between, which means that we are either eating to die - OR - Eating To LIVE !!!!
Energy is the Key to LIFE and we know that the Sun is the Source of all Energy, so if we focus on how to obtain as much Sun in the form of food as possible - the Key to Nutritional Health and Therapy.
Let us explore and examine Life Energy and how to obtain the best Quality and Value so that we may successfully manifest the Best out of Life and Enjoy a long, active and fruitful Life span!

Achieving and Maintaining Supreme Health and Fitness by increasing the level of Knowledge and Science of Life!

Peace
Sean Ali

CreateSpace eStore : https://www.createspace.com/7174743

OxyGen ... The Breath Of Life In Atomic Form!

Project Summary
Understanding Our Human Energy!: Energy Cycle & Transformation to Achieve Abundant LIFE!
Authored by Sean Ali

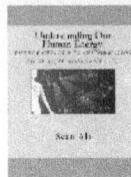

List Price: **$45.00**

8" x 10" (20.32 x 25.4 cm)
Full Color on White paper
224 pages

ISBN-13: 978-1546343462 (CreateSpace-Assigned)
ISBN-10: 1546343466
BISAC: Medical / Alternative Medicine

Peace and Blessings of Life!

•Do YOU Have health ailments/issues that YOU would like to over-come??
•Do YOU want to Improve the Quality of YOUR Life??
•Do YOU want to Experience and Enjoy ABUNDANT LIFE??
** Then this book is for YOU!

This small book is written so that we can explore and gain an Understanding of what our Human Energy System is, with a particular focus on What our Energy is, the Best sources and What to avoid to successfully Grow and LiVE so that we can Enjoy to the fullest, our GOD-Given potential of a Long and Abundant LIFE !!!!!!
Understanding our Human Energy is synonymous with Understanding our LIFE...it's what keeps us Alive and the main difference between Us and a body in the grave - Human Energy !!!!
Human Energy is manifested in the form of FOOD....Growing Our Own Food is the ONLY way that ensures we recieve the Highest Quality Life Energy - Straight from the Source!

OPEN THIS BOOK and Begin the neccessary steps to improve the Quality of YOUR LIFE!

Building and Maintaining Supreme Health & Fitness by increasing the level of Knowledge and Science of Life!

Peace!
Sean Ali, BS Health & Wellness

CreateSpace eStore: https://www.createspace.com/7126564

OxyGen ... The Breath Of Life In Atomic Form!

Project Summary
The Manual Of Healing Herbal Elements!: *Earth-based Solutions for Healing, Health & Life!
Authored by Sean Ali, Authored by Kareem Tyree, Authored by Gabriella Monique, Authored by Khalil Malik

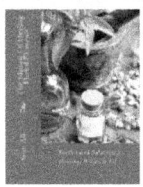

List Price: **$65.00**

8" x 10" (20.32 x 25.4 cm)
Full Color on White paper
336 pages

ISBN-13: 978-1547137985 (CreateSpace-Assigned)
ISBN-10: 1547137983
BISAC: Medical / Holistic Medicine

Peace and Blessings of Health!

This small work is being presented as a Manual of Healing, Health and Life. A comprehensive and scientific Handbook of Analysis and Research on over 80 Clinically & Commonly accessible Life & Healing Energy Herbal Elements. Each Herbal Element is categorized to include the latest research on the Uses, Actions, Dosages, Client Considerations, Contraindications & Interactions.

As many of Us are witnessing the RISE in Life-threatening dis-eases, especially in childhood Obesity and Diabetes, we are looking for more Natural ways to Heal

This Manual Of Healing is a Professional Grade handbook to Help YOU choose and use the BEST Naturally occurring Life Elements to Successfully Heal YourSelf!

We come from the Earth and ALL our Solutions come from the Earth!

PEACE!
Sean Ali

CreateSpace eStore: https://www.createspace.com/7225520

OxyGen ... The Breath Of Life In Atomic Form!

Project Summary
Understanding & Creating Herbal Healing!: Teas, Decoctions & Tinctures!
Authored by Sean Ali, Authored by Khalil Malik, Authored by Kareem Tyree, Authored by Gabriella Monique

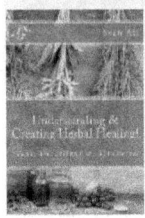

List Price: **$22.00**

7" x 10" (17.78 x 25.4 cm)
Full Color on White paper
108 pages

ISBN-13: **978-1548105457** (CreateSpace-Assigned)
ISBN-10: **1548105457**
BISAC: **Medical / Healing**

Peace and Blessings of Health!

This small work represents Volume 2 of my Science Of Healing Series and is being presented as a Handbook of Healing through the vehicles of Teas, Decoctions and Tinctures.

This is a comprehensive and scientific Handbook of Analysis and Research on over 30 Clinically used & easily accessible Life & Healing Energy Herbal Elements.

This Handbook Of Healing is Professional Grade and designed specifically to Help YOU choose and use the BEST Naturally occurring Life Elements to Successfully Heal YourSelf!
We come from the Earth and ALL our Solutions come from the Earth!

PEACE!
Sean Ali

CreateSpace eStore: https://www.createspace.com/7257513

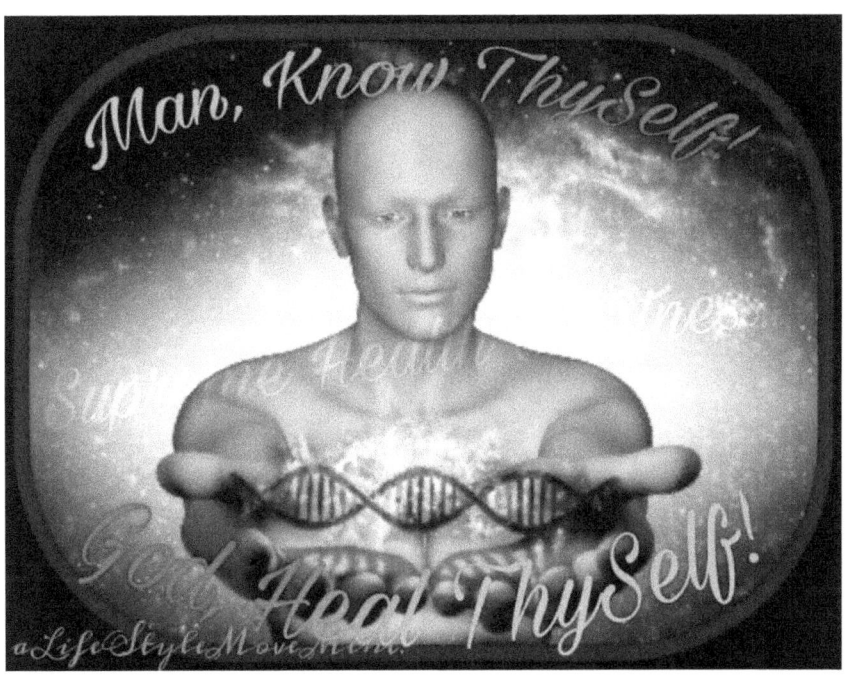

OxyGen ... The Breath Of Life In Atomic Form!

Achieving and Maintaing Supreme Health and Fitness by increasing the

Level of Knowlwdge and

Science of LIFE!!

www.ingramcontent.com/pod-product-compliance
Lightning Source LLC
Chambersburg PA
CBHW061437180526
45170CB00004B/1449